Advances in Geriatrics and Gerontology - Challenges of the New Millennium

Edited by Sara Palermo

Published in London, United Kingdom

Advances in Geriatrics and Gerontology - Challenges of the New Millennium
http://dx.doi.org/10.5772/intechopen.111024
Edited by Sara Palermo

Contributors
Alfi Syahri Pinem, Alina Crenguţa Nicolae, Anca Ungurianu, Anne Gibbone, Aulia Ulfa, Bonita Iravany Putri, Chiara Di Fazio, Cristina Manuela Drăgoi, Daniela Grădinaru, Denisa Margină, Devi Pahlawati, Elman Boy, Emilia Patricia Zarco, Hanna Matatyaho, Ion-Bogdan Dumitrescu, Ivando Adedra, Krisna Syahputra Hutapea, Milan Chang Gudjonsson, Mukulesh Gupta, Nishtha Manuja, Raudatul Popy Ramadani, Retno Pertiwi, Rika Karim Chan, Sara Palermo, Sunil Kumar, Tuhina Gupta, Ulil Amri Saragih

First published in London, United Kingdom, 2024 by IntechOpen
IntechOpen is the global imprint of INTECHOPEN LIMITED, registered in England and Wales, registration number: 11086078, 167-169 Great Portland Street, London, W1W 5PF, United Kingdom

British Library Cataloguing-in-Publication Data
A catalogue record for this book is available from the British Library

Additional hard and PDF copies can be obtained from orders@intechopen.com

Advances in Geriatrics and Gerontology - Challenges of the New Millennium
Edited by Sara Palermo
p. cm.
Print ISBN 978-1-83769-054-1
Online ISBN 978-1-83769-055-8
eBook (PDF) ISBN 978-1-83769-056-5

For EU product safety concerns:
IN TECH d.o.o., Prolaz Marije Krucifikse Kozulić 3, 51000 Rijeka, Croatia,
info@intechopen.com or visit our website at intechopen.com.

Meet the editor

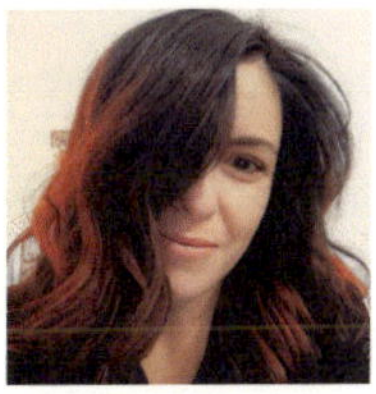

Sara Palermo has an MSc in Clinical Psychology and a Ph.D. in Experimental Neuroscience. She has been a researcher at the University of Turin, Italy, since 2022. She is specialized in neuropsychology and geriatrics and collaborates as a scientific consultant in the Neuroradiology Department, IRCCS Istituto Neurologico Carlo Besta, Italy. With expertise in multidimensional geriatric evaluations, neuroimaging meta-analysis, and advanced neuropsychological testing, Dr. Palermo contributes to *Frontiers in Psychology – Neuropsychology* as an assistant specialty chief editor.

Contents

Preface

At a time characterized by unprecedented global aging, the challenges posed by an aging population are great and underline the increasing importance of gerontological disciplines.

The world is experiencing a profound demographic shift, with older adults making up a growing proportion of the global population. This demographic shift brings with it a host of complex challenges, ranging from health care and social welfare to economic sustainability and public policy. With people living longer than ever before, innovative approaches to tackling age-related issues are urgently needed.

Against this background, the geriatric and gerontological disciplines are proving to be important pillars in tackling the complex problems of an aging society. Geriatrics, which deals with the medical and clinical aspects of aging, plays a central role in the specialized care of older adults, the treatment of age-related diseases, and the promotion of healthy aging. Gerontology, the multidisciplinary study of aging, encompasses various fields such as psychology, sociology, public health, and politics and offers comprehensive insights into the social, psychological, and environmental determinants of aging.

In the face of rapid demographic change and evolving healthcare needs, the relevance of geriatric and gerontological research and practice has never been greater. By fostering interdisciplinary collaboration, advancing scientific knowledge, and providing information for evidence-based interventions, these disciplines are instrumental in shaping policies and practices that promote the well-being and quality of life of older people worldwide.

Advances in Geriatrics and Gerontology – Challenges of the New Millennium represents a significant milestone in the ongoing dialogue on geriatric care and research. Indeed, this volume embodies the spirit of innovation and research that characterizes geriatric and gerontological research.

In these pages, you will embark on a journey through seven carefully crafted chapters, each offering a unique perspective on the multifaceted landscape of aging. From the winding paths of neuropsychology to the transformative potential of comprehensive geriatric assessments, physical activity interventions, and other critical topics, this volume encapsulates the breadth and depth of research in the field.

As editor, I would like to commend the dedication and expertise of our authors, whose invaluable insights have made this volume a cornerstone of the contemporary literature on geriatrics. Their tireless commitment to a better understanding of aging and its complex interrelationships is evident in the comprehensiveness of the topics covered.

I am committed to fostering interdisciplinary dialogue and promoting the dissemination of groundbreaking research findings. *Advances in Geriatrics and Gerontology – Challenges of the New Millennium* is an example of this commitment and serves as a catalyst for collaboration and innovation within the global scientific community.

My sincere thanks to the authors, reviewers, and editorial team whose combined efforts have made this publication possible.

I hope that this volume will stimulate further research, generate new ideas, and ultimately help to improve the quality of life of older people around the world.

Sara Palermo
Department of Psychology,
Interdepartmental Center for Advanced Studies in Neuroscience – NIT,
University of Turin,
Turin, Italy

Section 1

New Directions in Geriatrics and Gerontology

Chapter 1

Sirtuins and Melatonin: Linking Chronobiology to Inflammation and Aging

Anca Ungurianu, Cristina Manuela Drăgoi, Alina Crenguța Nicolae, Ion-Bogdan Dumitrescu, Daniela Grădinaru and Denisa Margină

Abstract

In recent years, the intricate interplay between sirtuins and melatonin has emerged as a fascinating area of research, with profound implications on various aspects of human health. This comprehensive chapter delves into the complex relationship between sirtuins and melatonin, as well as their essential roles in the regulation of circadian rhythms, inflammation, and aging. The attention is primarily directed to their impact on a range of critical health focal points, including cardiovascular diseases, central nervous system disorders, metabolic imbalances, musculoskeletal disorders, neoplasms, and the overarching process of aging, detailing all the complex biochemical mechanisms and physiological pathways that validate the intimately tailored functional relationship between the indoleamine hormone synthesized in the pinealocytes and the NAD^+-dependent histone deacetylases. These two components interact in complex ways, influencing processes such as cellular homeostasis, oxidative stress, and inflammatory cascade regulation. Age-related reductions in SIRT1 expression, influenced by melatonin levels, can deeply impact cellular functions. By elucidating the complex connections between sirtuins, melatonin, and chronobiological processes, we contribute to a deeper understanding of the fundamental mechanisms that trigger inflammation and aging-related diseases, and in the meantime underscore the promising avenues for future research and clinical interventions aimed at enhancing human health and extending the quality of life.

Keywords: sirtuin, melatonin, inflammation, aging, metabolic diseases

1. Introduction

Melatonin is mainly known for its involvement in sleep and circadian rhythm regulation, among other neuroendocrine processes [1], with reported anti-inflammatory, antioxidant, and antitumor effects [2, 3]. Melatonin is a hormone synthesized by the pineal gland that subsequently enters the bloodstream, enabling its distribution throughout various bodily systems. Moreover, it has the capability to penetrate the third ventricle of the brain *via* the pineal recess [4]. Melatonin receptors are mainly found throughout the central nervous system (CNS) and in immune cells, with various effects. Aside from its well-known role in circadian rhythm and sleep regulation, melatonin also acts as an anti-excitatory molecule in the CNS and is involved in the regulation of metabolic pathways, modulation of hormone secretion and of pro- and anti-inflammatory cytokines release, and it can even directly activate monocytes [4, 5]. Moreover, it maintains redox homeostasis by upregulating antioxidant enzymes, downregulating reactive oxygen- (ROS) and reactive nitrogen species (RNS)-generating enzymes, and also *via* its mitochondria-protective effects [4, 6–8].

Sirtuins are NAD^+-dependent enzymes with numerous physiological functions, regulating energy metabolism, inflammation, stress response, DNA repair, cell survival, and also being involved in circadian rhythms [9, 10]. Moreover, recent literature data links the sirtuin family to neurodegenerative, inflammation, and aging-associated diseases [11]. In humans, this enzyme family comprises seven isoforms, with different subcellular distribution and functions. Three enzymes are nuclear—SIRT1, SIRT6 and SIRT7, three mitochondrial—SIRT3, SIRT4, and SIRT5, and one cytosolic—SIRT2 [9]. However, SIRT1 often shuttles to the cytoplasm, while SIRT2 and SIRT3 can migrate to the nucleus, under certain conditions [9, 11]. The nuclear sirtuins are transcriptional and epigenetic regulators, stabilizing chromatin and deacetylating histones and non-histone proteins, such as transcriptional factors or DNA repair proteins [12–14]. They also modulate stress and oxidative stress response, maintain telomere integrity, and regulate apoptosis [9]. SIRT2 intervenes in several cellular processes, including cell cycle, apoptosis, DNA repair, metabolism, and senescence [11]. The mitochondrial sirtuins are mainly involved in metabolic regulation, energy metabolism, and mitochondrial function, maintaining redox and energy homeostasis [11].

Thus far, two sirtuin isoforms, SIRT1 and SIRT3, seem to be essential for the normal functioning of the circadian system, *via* multiple cellular pathways [4]. SIRT1 was established as a secondary mediator of melatonin's cellular actions, as numerous *in vivo* and *in vitro* studies confirmed its upregulation by melatonin [15]. Also, melatonin signaling in a SIRT1-mediated way is supported by the lack of melatonin effects in the case of SIRT1 inhibition or knockdown [16]. SIRT1 was reported to interact with the core circadian oscillator complex BMAL1:CLOCK (basic helix-loop-helix ARNT-like 1: circadian locomotor output cycles kaput), as to intervene in the positive feedback loop involving nicotinamide phosphoribosyltransferase (NAMPT) and nicotinamide adenine dinucleotide (NAD^+), influencing the expression of the period circadian regulator 2 (Per2) gene, a central player in circadian rhythm regulation [17–19]. SIRT3 can also intervene in the NAD^+ cycle, linking circadian rhythms to mitochondrial oxidative metabolism [20]. SIRT3 plays a pivotal role in mitochondrial antioxidant defense, increasing the expression of superoxide dismutase 2 (SOD 2) and catalase, two enzymes of paramount importance in counteracting the deleterious effects of oxidative stress [21, 22]. Moreover, intracellularly, melatonin is primarily concentrated in the mitochondria, its concentration in this organelle being higher than in any other [23]. Mitochondrial melatonin is not released in the systemic circulation and its synthesis is independent of light exposure [24]. Both melatonin and SIRT3 were reported to fight against oxidative stress by enhancing the expression of antioxidant enzymes [24–28], and melatonin's antioxidant effects seem to be SIRT3-mediated [29]. Consequently, its mitochondrial accumulation goes hand in hand with its antioxidant and antitumor actions, contributing to the maintenance of redox homeostasis and combatting malignant cell transformation [23].

Melatonin can act both as a pro-inflammatory and an anti-inflammatory molecule. This duality might come as a surprise, however, just as with other hormones, its function may vary under different conditions and when concerning various cell types [16, 30]. Its pro-inflammatory effect can be deemed beneficial when considering its action as an immune stimulatory agent concerning leukocytes and their ability to fight off pathogens [30–32] while proving detrimental in autoimmune maladies. The anti-inflammatory effects usually take center stage as they can be the basis of melatonin-based therapies in diseases with a low-grade inflammatory component, such as neurodegenerative or metabolic diseases, or characterized by high-grade inflammation, such as ischemia-reperfusion or brain injury and sepsis [16, 33, 34].

In this chapter, we aimed to construct a summary of the current state of understanding on a wide topic concerning the link between melatonin's effects and sirtuin signaling, concerning regulation of circadian rhythms, inflammation, and aging, in the most prevalent noncommunicable diseases currently associated with increased mortality and morbidity, selecting the most relevant, novel, and comprehensive research previously published by other scientists. The attention was primarily focused on their impact on cardiovascular diseases, central nervous system disorders, metabolic imbalances, neoplasms, and the process of aging, detailing the complex biochemical mechanisms involved.

2. Cardiovascular diseases

The imbalance of melatonin, which is one of the master regulators of the internal clocks in humans, is clearly associated with an increased risk of diseases, correlated with impaired sleep and aging-associated pathology, mainly cardiovascular, metabolic, and neurodegenerative disease [35–42].

One of the main pathways responsible for the correlation between melatonin and age-related chronic disease is represented by sirtuins [36, 37]. The interplay between the circadian machinery and sirtuins promotes cardiac health in a complex biochemistry of regulatory systems, mainly by modulating metabolic homeostasis and cell death or survival genes and influencing energy metabolism [43]. Recent research suggested that sirtuins in general, but SIRT1 in particular, have a crucial role in connecting the cellular metabolism to the circadian/internal clock [43, 44].

SIRT1 is directly implicated in the mechanistic development of cardiomyocytes, being responsible for regulating the voltage-gated cardiac sodium ion channels, reducing the risk of atherosclerotic plaque build-up, protection against oxidative damage, and lowering thrombotic risk [43, 45].

Melatonin is an amphiphilic molecule, so it can be found in all subcellular components, with a high concentration in cellular and subcellular membranes [8, 24, 46, 47]. As a result, it has the ability to act as a stabilizer of membrane processes acting against lipid peroxidation and oxidative impairment of mitochondrial DNA [28, 48, 49]. Melatonin is concentrated in the mitochondria and, as a consequence, it improves the electron transport chain efficiency and stimulates ATP production [50]. Its subcellular localization is somewhat overlapping with SIRT isoforms, supporting the intertwining of their signaling pathways; for example, recent data argues that melatonin and SIRT3 may act synergistically in regulating free radical generation and shielding mitochondria from oxidative damage [24].

Melatonin acts through different signaling pathways, either membrane- or organelle-focused, influencing the dynamics of physiological processes and protecting from pathological shifts. One of the key pathways modulated by melatonin concerning its protective actions is represented by modulating SIRT1 expression [9, 11]. Melatonin induces the transcriptional activation of nuclear factor erythroid 2-related factor 2 (Nrf2) and, consequently, antioxidant response element (ARE) through a SIRT1-dependent mechanism [51, 52]. Nrf2 is transcription factor that is able to bind to DNA and regulate the gene expression concerning antioxidant defense, as part of a master antioxidant and cytoprotective pathway, also inhibiting inflammation-enhancing signaling, such as the NLR family pyrin domain containing 3 (NLRP3) inflammasome [53–55].

Moreover, melatonin as well as its metabolites acts as ROS scavengers, stimulating the synthesis of antioxidant enzymes [7, 25, 28, 56]. Owing to its antioxidant action, melatonin was able to protect against ischemia-reperfusion injury in all organs, the activation sirtuins being most likely involved [10]. In a model of ischemia-reperfusion injury, the protective effects exerted by melatonin were dependent on the mitochondrial SIRT3. Melatonin's action was correlated with the stimulation of the adenosine monophosphate-activated kinase (AMPK)—peroxisome proliferator-activated receptor gamma coactivator 1-alpha (PGC-1α)—SIRT3 signaling, the activation of mitochondrial SOD and the enhancement of Nrf2 and mitochondrial transcription factor A (TFAM) expression [24, 57]. AMPK has a pivotal role in energy metabolism and homeostasis, adapting cell response to stress and nutrient availability. Recently, it was reported that AMPK functions as a redox sensor, also influencing autophagy, cell proliferation, and apoptosis, seemingly being involved in cardiovascular health and disease [58, 59]. PGC-1α is a key regulator of mitochondrial metabolism, being central to quite a few cellular pathways combating oxidative stress and inflammation [60]. This molecule is a crucial factor in the cellular stress response in the ischemic myocardium [60, 61]. TFAM is a mitochondrial DNA-binding protein vital for the maintenance of the mitochondrial genome, involved in the inflammatory stress response. An altered TFAM function was linked to pathological changes, especially in neurodegenerative diseases and aging [62, 63]. SIRT3 inhibition hinders mitochondrial SOD2 upregulation, leading to oxidative stress, which prevents melatonin's ability to protect the myocardium from free radical destruction [64].

Melatonin attenuates sepsis-induced myocardial injury by inhibiting caspase-3-induced apoptosis *via* SIRT1 activation [65]. Caspase-3 is a protease involved in tissue differentiation and regeneration, neural development, and, most famously, cell apoptosis, being possible target in the therapy of cardiovascular diseases, neurodegenerative disorders, and malignancies [66, 67]. Melatonin also exerts anti-inflammatory SIRT1-dependent effects, as the downregulation/inhibition of SIRT1 was reversed under the effect of melatonin in a H_2O_2-induced pro-inflammatory cell model [68]. On the other hand, experimental research shows that melatonin upregulates sirtuins, with a consequent downregulation of transcription for pro-inflammatory proteins and kappa-light-chain-enhancer of activated B cells (NF-κB) by suppressing the activation of toll-like receptor 4 (TLR4) and NLRP3 inflammasome [4, 69]. TLR4 activation leads to pro-inflammatory signaling (i.e., NF-κB) and synthesis of pro-inflammatory cytokines [70, 71]. NLRP3 inflammasome is a protein complex that assembles in response to cellular stress, promoting inflammation; its chronic aberrant activation is part of the etiopathogenesis of numerous diseases characterized by low-grade inflammation [72].

Furthermore, melatonin downregulates inflammation-associated enzymes such as inducible nitric oxide synthase (NOS) and cyclooxygenase 2 (COX-2), leading to lower levels of pro-inflammatory molecules, also contributing to an increase anti-inflammatory cytokines (e.g., interleukin 10, IL-10), thus exerting a protective effect against cardiovascular, metabolic, and autoimmune disease, which are all associated with oxidative stress and inflammation [73–76]. In a model of apolipoprotein E-deficient mice, melatonin decreased endothelial impairment, as well as the loss of SIRT1 and endothelial NOS activities, lowered tumor protein p53 and endothelin-1 expression. Administering melatonin formulated as a long-release dose and was more effective in counteracting endothelial dysfunction through multiple mechanisms, including SIRT modulation [46, 77].

Human studies confirm the correlation between melatonin, sirtuins, and the risk of cardiovascular disease. A clinical trial published in 2017 showed that the time of day (morning *vs.* afternoon) when patients underwent isolated aortic valve replacement interventions clearly influenced the overall survival, with a direct advantage of patients involved in afternoon intervention, who were characterized by fewer post-interventional events; also, that hypoxia-reoxygenation tolerance of the human myocardium is higher in the afternoon [35, 78]. These results confirm the observations regarding the higher incidence rate of cardiovascular events (myocardial infarction, stroke, arrhythmias, and sudden cardiac deaths) in the morning than in the evening. Also, from a chronotherapeutic perspective, the efficacy of antihypertensive treatments is higher when administered in the afternoon, according to both animal and human studies [41, 79–81].

There are several studies supporting the synergistic effects of melatonin and sirtuins, with cardiovascular beneficial outcome through antioxidant and anti-inflammatory mechanisms; in experimental/preclinical studies mimicking severe pathology, such as cardiac ischemia-reperfusion of normal and diabetic rats, endoplasmic reticulum stress in cardiomyocytes, lipopolysaccharide (LPS)-treated microglial cell lines, in brain injury by cecal ligation/puncture in mice, these results are confirmed [10, 51, 69, 82, 83]. This synergy is also supported by results showing that melatonin effects are antagonized by sirtuin inhibitors or by silencing the protein.

3. CNS disorders

CNS disorders encompass a wide variety of diseases from neurodegenerative diseases, such as Alzheimer's, Parkinson's, or multiple sclerosis, to neuropsychiatric disorders, such as depression, anxiety, or substance abuse, all being associated with a decreased quality of life [84–86]. Their etiopathogenesis is very complex, with multiple processes and alterations being involved, including neuroinflammation, disruption of autophagy, protein and lipid metabolism, redox, and energy and circadian homeostasis [86–88].

SIRT1 is widely expressed in the CNS, with anti-inflammatory and neuroprotective actions in numerous neurodegenerative diseases experimental models [1], and its recent link to melatonin signaling opens a new research path in the therapy of neurodegenerative diseases [89].

One of the mechanisms of melatonin's neuroprotective effect involves the increase of SIRT1 expression and the activation of SIRT1/Nrf2 pathway and the inhibition of the NLRP3 inflammasome [90, 91]. These might prove pivotal in the melatonin-based therapeutic approaches of some CNS disorders, seeing as the NLRP3 inflammasome is involved in the development or progression of neurodegenerative diseases [92], ischemia-reperfusion injury [93], traumatic brain injury [94], and cerebral tumors [95].

Neuroinflammation can be triggered by numerous factors, such as cellular damage or pathogens, and results into extracellular matrix damage and immunological reactions that can ultimately lead to neuronal oxidative damage and neurotransmitter dysfunction [1]. Further, the decrease in melatonin results in circadian dysregulation, decreased antioxidant defense, and alteration of normal mitochondrial functioning [26].

Inflammation is central to the pathogenesis of major depressive disorder (MMD) [91]. SIRT1 plays an important role in numerous cellular processes, including inflammation, in the hippocampus and central cortex [11], being recently linked to depression [96]. Mediation of inflammation by SIRT1, mainly *via* NF-κB and NLRP3 inflammasome downregulation, was shown to alleviate depression and anxiety-related behavioral deficits [91, 97, 98]. The NF-κB family of transcription factors is a key regulator of inflammation, immune responses, and cell proliferation, which, along with the NLRP3 inflammasome, contributes to amplifying inflammation [99–101].

Mitochondrial changes seem to play a crucial role in the development of MDD [26], and sirtuins are key regulators of mitochondrial processes, seeing as three of the seven family members are mitochondria-based [9]. The enhancement of the SIRT1–PGC-1α pathway is another signaling route *via* which melatonin exerts its protective effects, this time mitochondria being the main target, as PGC-1α is known as the master mitochondrial regulator, increasing their biogenesis and function [26]. SIRT1 enhancement by melatonin as a secondary signaling pathway [89] could correct some of the oxidative, mitochondrial, and neurotransmitter imbalances characteristic for depression and other neuropsychiatric disorders [102, 103], and contribute to uncovering more of the cellular pathways involved in melatonin's antidepressant-like effect [104, 105].

Neurodegenerative disease diagnosis had a sharp escalation in the last decades, increasing elderly morbidity and mortality [35]. Inflammation is part of normal aging; however, it is also part of the pathogenesis of several maladies, including neurodegenerative diseases [4]. This type of neuroinflammation is not of an infectious cause but entails moderate, slowly progressing microglia activation, supported by oxidative stress and mitochondria dysfunction, encompassing immune cells, astrocytes, and neurons [4].

Brain inflammation is a hallmark of neurodegenerative diseases, most notably Alzheimer's disease (AD) [4]. Both AD and Parkinson's disease (PD) are associated with an altered circadian rhythm, alongside impaired homeostasis of redox and inflammatory processes [4, 106]. AD is the most prevalent form of dementia in the elderly, being characterized by modified sleep patterns, abnormal melatonin secretion, and circadian dysregulation [26, 107, 108], shifting sleeping habits being reported early in its progression [35]. SIRT1 is an important link between circadian rhythm and redox homeostasis [35]. Melatonin is intimately linked to SIRT1 function in aging cells [109, 110]. Age-associated NAD^+ and SIRT1 deficiency, changes which are observed in neurodegenerative diseases also, are associated with mitochondrial dysfunction, autophagy, and circadian rhythm alterations, which can be reversed by melatonin [4, 111]. In preclinical and *in vitro* neurodegenerative diseases models, melatonin proved beneficial [112], while in clinical settings results varied [112], but the majority of studies reported improved sleep quality and reduced daytime sleepiness, stabilizing the circadian rhythm, and slowing down the progression of cognitive impairment [113–117].

Traumatic brain injury is a worldwide leading cause of mortality and morbidity, with debilitating long-term sequels. Sleep alterations are among the most common long-term post-injury implications. Animal studies showed that melatonin improved cognition as well as behavior; it also reduced post-injury cognitive decline and the risk of developing dementia, while human studies are scarce [118, 119]. The development of secondary injury following traumatic brain injury is dependent on the inflammatory response in the cerebral cortex, the NLRP3 inflammasome playing a central part [120–122]. SIRT1 was reported to have a protective role against traumatic brain injury, seeing as it mitigates oxidative stress and ROS production, which can, in turn, activate the NLRP3 inflammasome [1]. Further, resveratrol, a well-known SIRT1 activator [11], attenuated inflammation and oxidative stress by suppressing the NLRP3 inflammasome in a SIRT1-dependent manner [120]. Taking into consideration the melatonin-SIRT1 relationship, this neurohormone is a possible candidate as an additional therapeutic option in traumatic brain injury [118, 119].

4. Metabolic imbalances

Metabolic diseases, such as diabetes mellitus, metabolic syndrome, and obesity, have exponentially increased in the last decades, posing a serious threat to human health. They are characterized by inflammation and oxidative stress, along with impairments of cell metabolism, energy homeostasis, insulin secretion and function, and microbiota alterations [123–126].

Melatonin is involved in energy metabolism pathways and regulates epigenetic processes in neuronal cells, being biochemically interconnected with signaling pathways responsible for adjusting energy metabolism, such as insulin/insulin-like growth factor 1 (IGF-1), Forkhead box O (FoxO), and sirtuin pathways [110, 127–131]. Alterations of the expression and activity of circadian rhythm components are commonly found in patients with neurodegenerative, metabolic disorders, and cancer [37, 127, 132]. Also, melatonin levels and CLOCK expressions are reduced in patients with neurodegenerative and metabolic disorders [133–139].

All these pathological impairments have an underlying component of oxidative stress and mitochondrial function failure. Sirtuins, and especially SIRT1, as well as the peroxiredoxin protein family, are directly involved in the relationship between redox homeostasis and circadian rhythm, regulated by melatonin [37, 127, 132–139].

Metabolic syndrome and diabetes are associated with oxidative stress and inflammation, reunited under the umbrella of inflammaging, and would clearly benefit from the melatonin/SIRT synergy [69], seeing as melatonin is a key player in energy sensing/energy expenditure and body weight regulation. Animal studies showed that removing the pineal gland from rats led to a body weight increase that could be reversed by exogenous melatonin administration, along with a decrease of visceral fat; the results were found in animals fed either high fat or high fructose diets [140, 141]. Also, rat pinealectomy was associated with decreased insulin sensitivity and reduced glucose transporter type 4 (GLUT4) gene expression [142, 143]. In animal models, melatonin, as well as selective melatonin receptor agonists, induced a reduction of body weight and blood pressure, increased insulin sensitivity, and restored lipid homeostasis [34, 144]. These preclinical reports, among others [145, 146], highlight the potential of melatonin therapy in improving glucose metabolism and contribute to diabetes mellitus prevention [145, 146].

Impairments of melatonergic signaling due to genetic polymorphism support the development of a prediabetic status, type 2 diabetes, elevated cholesterol, triglycerides, and coronary heart disease; mice knocked out for the melatonin receptor MT1 or with pinealectomy exhibit insulin resistance [137, 142, 143, 147]. These metabolic alterations were reversed by melatonin, which decreased pro-inflammatory signaling (TNF-α, IL-1β) and inducible NOS by suppressing NF-κB expression in a SIRT-dependent manner [44, 148, 149].

Human studies confirm the metabolic protective action of melatonin, reporting antihyperlipidemic effects and a reduced insulin release (*via* pancreatic β-cells receptors), also contributing to alleviating metabolic syndrome *via* SIRT regulation, enhancing antioxidant and anti-inflammatory pathways [139, 150]. In type 2 diabetic patients low-circulating levels of melatonin were found, as well as increased mRNA for the melatonin membrane receptor [150, 151], while genetic variations of melatonin receptors are associated with impaired levels of fasting blood glucose and increased risk of type 2 diabetes, and also with polycystic ovary syndrome [45, 152–154]. Also, coronary artery disease patients show decreased melatonin levels; exogenous melatonin was effective in reducing blood pressure and cardiovascular rhythm alterations, preserving the availability of nitric oxide and yielding anti-remodeling cardiac effects, thus providing cardiovascular protection in metabolic syndrome patients [45, 137, 155]. Controlled clinical studies confirmed the antihypertensive properties of melatonin, and also underlined its ability to improve lipid profiles, with an increase of HDL, in metabolic syndrome patients [156].

5. Musculoskeletal disorders

Skeletal muscle is essential for posture and movement, but it is also directly involved in glucose uptake, thermal regulation, and nutritional balance, among other important physiological roles [157–159]. Therefore, deterioration of skeletal muscle mass is associated with impaired glucose homeostasis, and not only with posture/movement-associated difficulties (falls, fractures, disability) [160]. Moreover, skeletal muscle ailments are considerably increasing in aging, thus bringing up the costs of healthcare and having a negative impact on the quality of life [159].

Melatonin was reported to support muscle activity through its ability to maintain mitochondrial function, alongside oxidative stress reduction and inhibition of cardiolipin peroxidation [15, 24, 69]. Cardiolipin is a dimeric phospholipid found in the inner mitochondrial membrane that undergoes oxidation and translocation to the cytosolic side of the outer mitochondrial membrane under oxidative stress conditions, signaling a dysfunctional mitochondria [161, 162]. In Refs., [163, 164] dystrophic muscle diseases are biochemically characterized by inflammation, redox imbalance, and mitochondrial dysfunction, and could benefit from melatonin treatment [160, 165]. This is attributable to its lipophilic nature, making it possible to pass through cells and mitochondrial membranes and the blood-brain barrier, as well as its effect as a calcium homeostasis regulator during muscle contraction [166, 167]. When administered as a nutraceutical in preclinical, but also in clinical studies, it improved muscle metabolism and strength [163, 164]. These positive effects are also pointed out in age-related sarcopenia and muscle weakness [160].

Chronic melatonin administration in rat and mouse models of muscle injury reduced apoptosis, increased twitch force, and accelerated the regeneration of satellite cells. Women with fibromyalgia benefit from melatonin administration which induces reduction of symptoms such as chronic muscular pain, cognitive dysfunctions, and sleep disorders [159, 168, 169].

Calpain is a receptor of calcium, found in the cytoplasm of skeletal muscle cells in an inactive form, being controlled by intracellular calcium ion concentration and calpain inhibitory protein. An increase in the skeletal muscle cells' cytoplasmic Ca^{2+} concentration activates calpain, resulting in the hydrolysis of skeletal muscle fibers, leading to reduced contractility. Melatonin was reported to inhibit calpain, but more in-depth studies are required to establish its clinical potential [170–172].

In Refs., [159, 168, 169] literature data reveal melatonin to be a promising agent for muscle regeneration and maintenance, with a possible use in chronic diseases, especially those associated with aging, sirtuins being just one of the signaling pathways involved. Nevertheless, further studies, both preclinical and clinical, are needed to establish its muscle-protective mechanisms and clinical use aspects.

6. Neoplasms

Malignancies have an ever-increasing prevalence and a cancer diagnosis has a severe impact on the quality of life and mental well-being of patients [173]. The antitumor effect of melatonin was reported in different types of cancer, interfering with various cancer hallmarks, mitigating cancer initiation, progression, and metastasis [174, 175].

The disruption of circadian rhythm due to exposure to excessive light or frequent long-distance travel entails an alteration of melatonin synthesis and secretion, with an associated increased risk of cancer development [176, 177]. *In vitro* studies in breast cancer cells showed that exposure to white fluorescent light led to decreased melatonin levels and increased tumor growth [178], while the blood of volunteers exposed to white fluorescent light during nighttime had lower melatonin levels and proved a better tumor growth medium [178].

Melatonin administration decreased proliferation parameters and induced a reduction in tumor growth, concomitantly downregulating SIRT1 [179]. The downregulation or inhibition of SIRT1 led to increased pro-oxidant and antitumor activity [180, 181], while its activation decreased melatonin's anticancer action [182].

The relationship between SIRT1 and melatonin in cancer cells is opposite to that in nontumor cells, melatonin acting as an inhibitor of SIRT1 activity [44]. This might come as a surprise, but seeing as SIRT1 is overexpressed in some types of cancer [183, 184], a context-specific role for melatonin in regulating the activity of this sirtuin is plausible [185]. The dual role of melatonin concerning SIRT1 regulation in normal and malignant cells seems to entail its ability to either stimulate or inhibit the activity of SIRT1. Moreover, this regulation might not only target cell proliferation but also the control of circadian regulation genes, such as BMAL1 or Per2, which are key players in maintaining tissue homeostasis [90, 185].

7. Aging

Aging is a ubiquitous phenomenon that encompasses numerous biological changes that, in time, lead to the decline of an organism [186]. In humans, aging entails a gradual accumulation of physical and cognitive alterations, with an increased risk of developing various maladies, such as cardiovascular, metabolic, or neurodegenerative diseases and malignancies [186–188]. These often cause a marked decline in the quality of life, being associated with higher morbidity and mortality.

Aging is associated with an alteration of circadian rhythm synchrony and reduced secretion of melatonin [1, 35]. Also, a reduction of SIRT1 activity was observed in senescence, while its inhibition abolished a number of melatonin's cellular effects [69]. Lower SIRT1 levels were observed in the suprachiasmatic nucleus (SCN) of aging mice, affecting the functioning of the core circadian oscillator BMAL1:CLOCK, while its overexpression prevented aging-depending circadian rhythm alterations and its silencing in young animals decreased BMAL1 and Per2 gene expression [189].

Low-grade inflammation is a major component of physiological aging, especially considering its association with the alteration of brain function, neurodegeneration, and mood disorders [137, 190]. The contribution of inflammation to the aging process is known as inflammaging [4, 16]. Apart from playing a central role in longevity, regulating cellular processes as cell cycle, apoptosis, or DNA repair, SIRT1 is involved in modulating antioxidant and anti-inflammatory processes [11]. SIRT1 seems to be an important factor in trying to assess the extent of melatonin's effects on aging and aging-associated low-grade inflammation [1]. Moreover, melatonin enhances the antioxidant defense of senescent cells, regulating redox homeostasis. A central player in this effect is SIRT1, whose upregulation results in the increased expression of antioxidants *via* Nrf2 and FOXO pathways, modulating mitochondrial ROS production and autophagy, while inhibiting NF-κB signaling [35].

Despite all these, some conflicting results regarding the effect of melatonin treatment on SIRT2 activity were reported in preclinical models of aging. One research group found no effect on SIRT2 in neurons from the dentate gyrus [191], while another group observed that melatonin treatment led to a decrease in SIRT2 activity in the hippocampus of adult rats [192], and in the colon and hippocampus of aged rats [193, 194], reducing oxidative stress parameters and pro-apoptotic proteins.

Both the pro-inflammatory effect of melatonin, as well as the anti-inflammatory, must be considered when addressing its potential use in mitigating some aging-associated signs and symptoms [69]. Most data are supportive of its beneficial, anti-inflammatory actions. However, some reports concerning autoimmune diseases, such as rheumatoid arthritis or multiple sclerosis, bring to the fore its possible detrimental effects [195–197]. Its protective actions fall mainly under the umbrella of the above-mentioned and well-documented antioxidant and anti-inflammatory effects, along with its stimulation of the immune system, promoting healing and maintaining homeostasis [187, 188, 198, 199]. A special melatonin-mediated pathway, central to the aging process, is the enhancement of SIRT1 activity.

8. Discussion

Melatonin, a hormone primarily synthesized in the pineal gland, has emerged as a critical regulator of circadian rhythms and a multifunctional molecule with antioxidant, anti-inflammatory, and neuroprotective properties, involving numerous cellular signaling pathways (**Figure 1**).

The anti-inflammatory activity of melatonin involves both immunological and non-immunological processes [16]. The latter mainly includes protection against oxidative stress by promoting antioxidant defense and decreasing the formation of reactive oxygen and nitrogen species, and the preventing mitochondrial dysfunction [16]. It contributes to an anti-inflammatory pathway involving sirtuin activation, namely SIRT1, Nrf2 upregulation, and nuclear factor NF-κB downregulation [1, 69]. Also, it was reported to downregulate COX-2 and neuronal NOS, to prevent TLR4 and NLRP3 inflammasome activation [16]. These resulted in an increased secretion of anti-inflammatory cytokines and decreased production of ROS and pro-inflammatory cytokines [1, 16].

Exploring the melatonin-sirtuins interaction holds significant promise in advancing our understanding of their joint impact on human health. On the other hand, sirtuins, a family of deacetylase enzymes, play fundamental roles in cellular processes such as gene expression, DNA repair, and stress response. The interplay between melatonin and sirtuins has been implicated in a spectrum of biological phenomena, ranging from circadian rhythm regulation to cellular homeostasis and physiological aging. Investigating the intricate crosstalk between melatonin and sirtuins has the potential to unlock novel insights into the mechanisms governing these processes and different pathological *milieu* modulation.

Moreover, understanding how melatonin influences sirtuins activity and *vice versa* could pave the way for the development of innovative therapeutic strategies targeting a wide array of health conditions, including sleep disorders, cardiovascular and metabolic diseases, neurodegenerative disorders, and cancer. These melatonin-sirtuins studies not only shed light on the fundamental principles of circadian biology and cellular physiology but also offer promising avenues for enhancing human health and well-being.

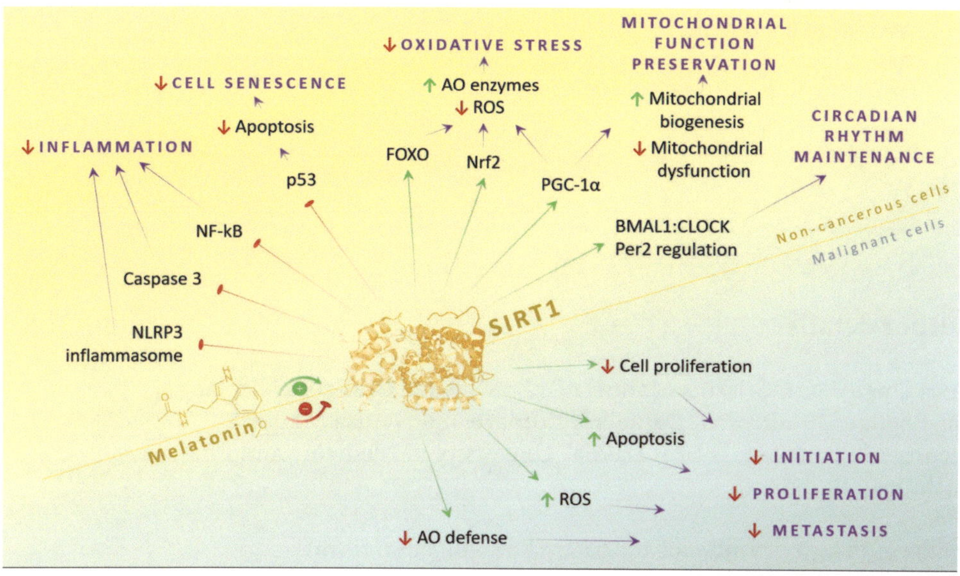

Figure 1.
An overview of the SIRT1-mediated melatonin effects in noncancerous and malignant cells. ROS-reactive oxygen species, AO-antioxidant, BMAL1:CLOCK-basic helix-loop-helix ARNT-like 1: circadian locomotor output cycles kaput, Per2-period circadian regulator 2 gene, PGC-1α-peroxisome proliferator-activated receptor gamma coactivator 1-alpha, Nrf2-nuclear factor erythroid 2-related factor 2, FOXO-Forkhead box O, NF-κB-kappa-light-chain-enhancer of activated B cells, NLRP3-NLR family pyrin domain containing 3 inflammasome.

9. Outlook

Melatonin is considered one of the master regulators of the circadian rhythm, being intensively studied for its pleiotropic effects concerning redox imbalance, inflammation, immune response, aging, cell proliferation, and even fertility. The present chapter aims to critically analyze the latest scientific information regarding the interplay between sirtuins and melatonin in order to better understand the role of this complex system and its potential modulation in preventing/treating various afflictions. As a result, we pointed out that sirtuin signaling is directly involved in the cardio- and neuroprotective effects attributed to melatonin, as well as its ability to support musculoskeletal function and regeneration and to restore metabolic and energy homeostasis. Regarding malignancies, the relationship between SIRT1 and melatonin in cancer cells is opposite to that in non-tumor cells, with an overall antitumor action. All these reported effects are integrated as important pathways, justifying the protective effect of melatonin in aging-associated pathology through SIRT-mediated pathways. In this complex picture, there is an acute need for further studies to substantiate all these scientific claims, since there is a great imbalance between *in vitro*, preclinical and clinical studies, for each of the above-mentioned effects. Also, a systematic review of the latest literature data, encompassing the cellular pathways through which melatonin modulates physio-pathological processes, focusing on the interconnection with sirtuins, is highly needed considering the current heterogeneous research output.

Conflict of interest

The authors declare no conflict of interest.

Author details

Anca Ungurianu, Cristina Manuela Drăgoi*, Alina Crenguța Nicolae, Ion-Bogdan Dumitrescu, Daniela Grădinaru and Denisa Margină
Faculty of Pharmacy, "Carol Davila" University of Medicine and Pharmacy, Bucharest, Romania

*Address all correspondence to: cristina.dragoi@umfcd.ro

References

[1] Chen H et al. Involvement of the SIRT1-NLRP3 pathway in the inflammatory response. Cell Communication and Signaling: CCS. 2023;**21**(1):185

[2] Tordjman S et al. Melatonin: Pharmacology, functions and therapeutic benefits. Current Neuropharmacology. 2017;**15**(3):434-443

[3] Zhou H et al. Melatonin suppresses platelet activation and function against cardiac ischemia/reperfusion injury via PPARgamma/FUNDC1/mitophagy pathways. Journal of Pineal Research. 2017;**63**(4)

[4] Hardeland R et al. Melatonin and brain inflammaging. Progress in Neurobiology. 2015;**127-128**:46-63

[5] Hardeland R. Melatonin and the theories of aging: A critical appraisal of melatonin's role in antiaging mechanisms. Journal of Pineal Research. 2013;**55**(4):325-356

[6] Drăgoi CM, Nicolae AC, editors. Melatonin - Molecular Biology, Clinical and Pharmaceutical Approaches. IntechOpen. 2018. DOI: 10.5772/intechopen.74993

[7] Galano A, Tan DX, Reiter RJ. On the free radical scavenging activities of melatonin's metabolites, AFMK and AMK. Journal of Pineal Research. 2013;**54**(3):245-257

[8] Menendez-Pelaez A, Reiter RJ. Distribution of melatonin in mammalian tissues: The relative importance of nuclear versus cytosolic localization. Journal of Pineal Research. 1993;**15**(2):59-69

[9] Ungurianu A, Zanfirescu A, Margina D. Regulation of gene expression through food-curcumin as a Sirtuin activity modulator. Plants (Basel). 2022;**11**(13)

[10] Yu L et al. Melatonin receptor-mediated protection against myocardial ischemia/reperfusion injury: Role of SIRT1. Journal of Pineal Research. 2014;**57**(2):228-238

[11] Ungurianu A, Zanfirescu A, Margina D. Sirtuins, resveratrol and the intertwining cellular pathways connecting them. Ageing Research Reviews. 2023;**88**:101936

[12] Toiber D, Sebastian C, Mostoslavsky R. Characterization of nuclear sirtuins: Molecular mechanisms and physiological relevance. Handbook of Experimental Pharmacology. 2011;**206**:189-224

[13] Soetikno V et al. Curcumin prevents diabetic cardiomyopathy in streptozotocin-induced diabetic rats: Possible involvement of PKC-MAPK signaling pathway. European Journal of Pharmaceutical Sciences. 2012;**47**(3):604-614

[14] Houtkooper RH, Pirinen E, Auwerx J. Sirtuins as regulators of metabolism and healthspan. Nature Reviews. Molecular Cell Biology. 2012;**13**(4):225-238

[15] Hardeland R. Melatonin and the pathologies of weakened or dysregulated circadian oscillators. Journal of Pineal Research. 2017;**62**(1)

[16] Hardeland R. Melatonin and inflammation-story of a double-edged blade. Journal of Pineal Research. 2018;**65**(4):e12525

[17] Ramsey KM et al. Circadian clock feedback cycle through

NAMPT-mediated NAD+ biosynthesis. Science. 2009;**324**(5927):651-654

[18] Nakahata Y et al. Circadian control of the NAD+ salvage pathway by CLOCK-SIRT1. Science. 2009;**324**(5927):654-657

[19] Imai S. "Clocks" in the NAD world: NAD as a metabolic oscillator for the regulation of metabolism and aging. Biochimica et Biophysica Acta. 2010;**1804**(8):1584-1590

[20] Peek CB et al. Circadian clock NAD+ cycle drives mitochondrial oxidative metabolism in mice. Science. 2013;**342**(6158):1243417

[21] Tao R et al. Sirt3-mediated deacetylation of evolutionarily conserved lysine 122 regulates MnSOD activity in response to stress. Molecular Cell. 2010;**40**(6):893-904

[22] Rangarajan P et al. Sirtuin 3 regulates Foxo3a-mediated antioxidant pathway in microglia. Neuroscience. 2015;**311**:398-414

[23] Reiter RJ et al. Melatonin: A mitochondrial resident with a diverse skill set. Life Sciences. 2022;**301**:120612

[24] Reiter RJ et al. Melatonin mitigates mitochondrial meltdown: Interactions with SIRT3. International Journal of Molecular Sciences. 2018;**19**(8)

[25] Allegra M et al. The chemistry of melatonin's interaction with reactive species. Journal of Pineal Research. 2003;**34**(1):1-10

[26] Anderson G. Linking the biological underpinnings of depression: Role of mitochondria interactions with melatonin, inflammation, sirtuins, tryptophan catabolites, DNA repair and oxidative and nitrosative stress, with consequences for classification and cognition. Progress in Neuro-Psychopharmacology & Biological Psychiatry. 2018;**80**(Pt C):255-266

[27] Drăgoi CM, Nicolae AC. Introductory Chapter: Melatonin, the Integrative Molecule within the Human Architecture. Melatonin - Molecular Biology, Clinical and Pharmaceutical Approaches. IntechOpen. 2018. DOI: 10.5772/intechopen.81071

[28] Garcia JJ et al. Protective effects of melatonin in reducing oxidative stress and in preserving the fluidity of biological membranes: A review. Journal of Pineal Research. 2014;**56**(3):225-237

[29] Chen Y et al. Melatonin protects hepatocytes against bile acid-induced mitochondrial oxidative stress via the AMPK-SIRT3-SOD2 pathway. Free Radical Research. 2015;**49**(10):1275-1284

[30] Drăgoi CM et al. In vitro effects of some bio-indoles on the transmembrane potential of Jurkat E6. 1 limphoblasts. Farmácia. 2012;**60**(2):240-248

[31] Carrillo-Vico A et al. Melatonin: Buffering the immune system. International Journal of Molecular Sciences. 2013;**14**(4):8638-8683

[32] Carrillo-Vico A et al. A review of the multiple actions of melatonin on the immune system. Endocrine. 2005;**27**(2):189-200

[33] Nicolae AC et al. In vitro P-GP expression after administration of CNS active drugs. Farmácia. 2016;**64**(6):844-850

[34] Dragoi CM et al. Characteristics of glucose homeostasis and lipidic profile in a hamster metabolic syndrome model, after the co-administration of melatonin and Irbesartan in a multiparticulate pharmaceutical

formation. In: 2nd International Conference on Interdisciplinary Management of Diabetes Mellitus and its Complications, Interdiab 2016. Romania: Bucharest; 2016

[35] Yanar K, Simsek B, Cakatay U. Integration of melatonin related redox homeostasis, aging, and circadian rhythm. Rejuvenation Research. 2019;**22**(5):409-419

[36] Reiter RJ. Pineal melatonin: Cell biology of its synthesis and of its physiological interactions. Endocrine Reviews. 1991;**12**(2):151-180

[37] Salminen A, Kaarniranta K, Kauppinen A. Crosstalk between oxidative stress and SIRT1: Impact on the aging process. International Journal of Molecular Sciences. 2013;**14**(2):3834-3859

[38] Dragoi CM, Andreea LA, Cristina ED-P, Ion BD, Daniela EP, George TA, et al. Melatonin: A Silent Regulator of the Glucose Homeostasis. Carbohydrate. InTech. 2017. DOI: 10.5772/66625

[39] Drăgoi CM et al. 1 cell line studies regarding the effects of some bio-indoles on the membrane fluidity. Farmácia. 2012;**60**(1):13-20

[40] Nicolae AC et al. Clinical implications of the indolergic system and oxidative stress in physiological gestational homeostasis. Farmácia. 2015;**63**(1):46-51

[41] Nicolae AC et al. Chronotherapy Advances in the Management of Chronic Neurological and Cardiovascular Diseases: Complex Interactions of Circadian Rhythm Environmental Inputs, Nutrition and Drug Administration and their Impact on Human Health, in Circadian Rhythm-New Insights into Physiological and Pathological Implications. London: IntechOpen; 2022

[42] Stanciu AE et al. Clinical significance of serum melatonin in predicting the severity of oral squamous cell carcinoma. Oncology Letters. 2020;**19**(2):1537-1543

[43] Soni SK et al. Sirtuins and the circadian clock interplay in cardioprotection: Focus on sirtuin 1. Cellular and Molecular Life Sciences. 2021;**78**(6):2503-2515

[44] Jung-Hynes B, Reiter RJ, Ahmad N. Sirtuins, melatonin and circadian rhythms: Building a bridge between aging and cancer. Journal of Pineal Research. 2010;**48**(1):9-19

[45] Song YJ, Zhong CB, Wu W. Cardioprotective effects of melatonin: Focusing on its roles against diabetic cardiomyopathy. Biomedicine & Pharmacotherapy. 2020;**128**:110260

[46] Ramis MR et al. Caloric restriction, resveratrol and melatonin: Role of SIRT1 and implications for aging and related-diseases. Mechanisms of Ageing and Development. 2015;**146-148**:28-41

[47] Costa EJ, Lopes RH, Lamy-Freund MT. Permeability of pure lipid bilayers to melatonin. Journal of Pineal Research. 1995;**19**(3):123-126

[48] Karbownik M et al. Renal toxicity of the carcinogen delta-aminolevulinic acid: Antioxidant effects of melatonin. Cancer Letters. 2000;**161**(1):1-7

[49] Drăgoi C et al. DNA targeting AS a molecular mechanism underlying endogenous indoles biological effects. Farmácia. 2019;**67**(2)

[50] Acuna-Castroviejo D et al. Characterization of high-affinity melatonin binding sites in purified cell

nuclei of rat liver. Journal of Pineal Research. 1994;**16**(2):100-112

[51] Shah SA et al. Melatonin stimulates the SIRT1/Nrf2 Signaling pathway counteracting lipopolysaccharide (LPS)-induced oxidative stress to rescue postnatal rat brain. CNS Neuroscience & Therapeutics. 2017;**23**(1):33-44

[52] Ding YW et al. SIRT1 exerts protective effects against paraquat-induced injury in mouse type II alveolar epithelial cells by deacetylating NRF2 in vitro. International Journal of Molecular Medicine. 2016;**37**(4):1049-1058

[53] Gureev AP, Popov VN, Starkov AA. Crosstalk between the mTOR and Nrf2/ARE signaling pathways as a target in the improvement of long-term potentiation. Experimental Neurology. 2020;**328**:113285

[54] Ghareghomi S et al. Nrf2 modulation in breast cancer. Biomedicine. 2022;**10**(10)

[55] Ahmed SM et al. Nrf2 signaling pathway: Pivotal roles in inflammation. Biochimica et Biophysica Acta - Molecular Basis of Disease. 2017;**1863**(2):585-597

[56] Fischer TW et al. Melatonin as a major skin protectant: From free radical scavenging to DNA damage repair. Experimental Dermatology. 2008;**17**(9):713-730

[57] Yu L et al. Melatonin ameliorates myocardial ischemia/reperfusion injury in type 1 diabetic rats by preserving mitochondrial function: Role of AMPK-PGC-1alpha-SIRT3 signaling. Scientific Reports. 2017;**7**:41337

[58] Wu S, Zou MH. AMPK, mitochondrial function, and cardiovascular disease. International Journal of Molecular Sciences. 2020;**21**(14)

[59] Wang S, Song P, Zou MH. AMP-activated protein kinase, stress responses and cardiovascular diseases. Clinical Science (London, England). 2012;**122**(12):555-573

[60] Aggarwal R et al. Novel therapeutic approaches enhance PGC1-alpha to reduce oxidant stress-inflammatory Signaling and improve functional recovery in hibernating myocardium. Antioxidants (Basel). 2022;**11**(11)

[61] Butterick TA et al. Pioglitazone increases PGC1-alpha signaling within chronically ischemic myocardium. Basic Research in Cardiology. 2016;**111**(3):37

[62] Mposhi A et al. Regulation of mitochondrial gene expression, the epigenetic enigma. Frontiers in Bioscience (Landmark edition). 2017;**22**(7):1099-1113

[63] Kang I, Chu CT, Kaufman BA. The mitochondrial transcription factor TFAM in neurodegeneration: Emerging evidence and mechanisms. FEBS Letters. 2018;**592**(5):793-811

[64] Zhai M et al. Melatonin ameliorates myocardial ischemia reperfusion injury through SIRT3-dependent regulation of oxidative stress and apoptosis. Journal of Pineal Research. 2017;**63**(2)

[65] Liu Y et al. Melatonin: A potential adjuvant therapy for septic myopathy. Biomedicine & Pharmacotherapy. 2023;**158**:114209

[66] Shalini S et al. Old, new and emerging functions of caspases. Cell Death and Differentiation. 2015;**22**(4):526-539

[67] Asadi M et al. Caspase-3: Structure, function, and biotechnological aspects. Biotechnology and Applied Biochemistry. 2022;**69**(4):1633-1645

[68] Lim HD et al. Cytoprotective and anti-inflammatory effects of melatonin in hydrogen peroxide-stimulated CHON-001 human chondrocyte cell line and rabbit model of osteoarthritis via the SIRT1 pathway. Journal of Pineal Research. 2012;**53**(3):225-237

[69] Hardeland R. Aging, melatonin, and the pro- and anti-inflammatory networks. International Journal of Molecular Sciences. 2019;**20**(5)

[70] Vaure C, Liu Y. A comparative review of toll-like receptor 4 expression and functionality in different animal species. Frontiers in Immunology. 2014;**5**:316

[71] Li Y, Jiang Q, Wang L. Appetite regulation of TLR4-induced inflammatory signaling. Frontiers in Endocrinology. 2021;**12**:777997

[72] Sharma BR, Kanneganti TD. NLRP3 inflammasome in cancer and metabolic diseases. Nature Immunology. 2021;**22**(5):550-559

[73] Chattree V et al. A comprehensive review on modulation of SIRT1 signaling pathways in the immune system of COVID-19 patients by phytotherapeutic melatonin and epigallocatechin-3-gallate. Journal of Food Biochemistry. 2022;**46**(12):e14259

[74] Martin Gimenez VM et al. New proposal involving nanoformulated melatonin targeted to the mitochondria as a potential COVID-19 treatment. Nanomedicine (London, England). 2020;**15**(29):2819-2821

[75] Niu Z, Li R. Clinical study of novel coronavirus pneumonia prevention by melatonin. Reproductive Biomedicine Online. 2020;**41**(6):1156

[76] Ozturk G, Akbulut KG, Guney S. Melatonin, aging, and COVID-19: Could melatonin be beneficial for COVID-19 treatment in the elderly? Turkish Journal of Medical Sciences. 2020;**50**(6):1504-1512

[77] Rodella LF et al. Aging and vascular dysfunction: Beneficial melatonin effects. Age (Dordrecht, Netherlands). 2013;**35**(1):103-115

[78] Montaigne D et al. Daytime variation of perioperative myocardial injury in cardiac surgery and its prevention by Rev-Erbalpha antagonism: A single-Centre propensity-matched cohort study and a randomised study. Lancet. 2018;**391**(10115):59-69

[79] Kuehn BM. The Heart's circadian rhythms point to potential treatment strategies. Circulation. 2016;**134**(23):1907-1908

[80] Martino TA et al. The primary benefits of angiotensin-converting enzyme inhibition on cardiac remodeling occur during sleep time in murine pressure overload hypertrophy. Journal of the American College of Cardiology. 2011;**57**(20):2020-2028

[81] Zairi I et al. Effect of intermittent fasting and chronotherapy on blood pressure control in hypertensive patients during Ramadan. Arterial Hypertension. 2022;**26**(2):67-72

[82] Yu L et al. Reduced silent information regulator 1 signaling exacerbates myocardial ischemia-reperfusion injury in type 2 diabetic rats and the protective effect of melatonin. Journal of Pineal Research. 2015;**59**(3):376-390

[83] Zhao L et al. Melatonin alleviates brain injury in mice subjected to

cecal ligation and puncture via attenuating inflammation, apoptosis, and oxidative stress: The role of SIRT1 signaling. Journal of Pineal Research. 2015;**59**(2):230-239

[84] Zschucke E, Gaudlitz K, Strohle A. Exercise and physical activity in mental disorders: Clinical and experimental evidence. Journal of Preventive Medicine and Public Health. 2013;**46**(Suppl. 1):S12-S21

[85] Mihai DP et al. Effects of venlafaxine, risperidone and Febuxostat on Cuprizone-induced demyelination, Behavioral deficits and oxidative stress. International Journal of Molecular Sciences. 2021;**22**(13)

[86] Bogie JFJ et al. Fatty acid metabolism in the progression and resolution of CNS disorders. Advanced Drug Delivery Reviews. 2020;**159**:198-213

[87] Nassan M, Videnovic A. Circadian rhythms in neurodegenerative disorders. Nature Reviews. Neurology. 2022;**18**(1):7-24

[88] Haidar M et al. Lipophagy: A new player in CNS disorders. Trends in Endocrinology and Metabolism. 2021;**32**(11):941-951

[89] Hardeland R. Melatonin and microglia. International Journal of Molecular Sciences. 2021;**22**(15)

[90] Mayo JC et al. Melatonin and sirtuins: A "not-so unexpected" relationship. Journal of Pineal Research. 2017;**62**(2)

[91] Arioz BI et al. Melatonin attenuates LPS-induced acute depressive-like Behaviors and microglial NLRP3 Inflammasome activation through the SIRT1/Nrf2 pathway. Frontiers in Immunology. 2019;**10**:1511

[92] Hanslik KL, Ulland TK. The role of microglia and the Nlrp3 Inflammasome in Alzheimer's disease. Frontiers in Neurology. 2020;**11**:570711

[93] Minutoli L et al. ROS-mediated NLRP3 Inflammasome activation in brain, heart, kidney, and testis ischemia/reperfusion injury. Oxidative Medicine and Cellular Longevity. 2016;**2016**:2183026

[94] Liu HD et al. Expression of the NLRP3 inflammasome in cerebral cortex after traumatic brain injury in a rat model. Neurochemical Research. 2013;**38**(10):2072-2083

[95] Li L, Liu Y. Aging-related gene signature regulated by Nlrp3 predicts glioma progression. American Journal of Cancer Research. 2015;**5**(1):442-449

[96] Lei Y et al. SIRT1 in forebrain excitatory neurons produces sexually dimorphic effects on depression-related behaviors and modulates neuronal excitability and synaptic transmission in the medial prefrontal cortex. Molecular Psychiatry. 2020;**25**(5):1094-1111

[97] Abe-Higuchi N et al. Hippocampal sirtuin 1 signaling mediates depression-like behavior. Biological Psychiatry. 2016;**80**(11):815-826

[98] Fan J et al. SIRT1 mediates Apelin-13 in ameliorating chronic normobaric hypoxia-induced anxiety-like behavior by suppressing NF-kappaB pathway in mice hippocampus. Neuroscience. 2018;**381**:22-34

[99] Wu JT, Kral JG. The NF-kappaB/IkappaB signaling system: A molecular target in breast cancer therapy. The Journal of Surgical Research. 2005;**123**(1):158-169

[100] Mitchell S, Vargas J, Hoffmann A. Signaling via the NFkappaB system.

Wiley Interdisciplinary Reviews. Systems Biology and Medicine. 2016;**8**(3):227-241

[101] Dolcet X et al. NF-kB in development and progression of human cancer. Virchows Archiv. 2005;**446**(5):475-482

[102] Rajkhowa B et al. Activation of SIRT-1 signalling in the prevention of bipolar disorder and related Neurocomplications: Target activators and influences on neurological dysfunctions. Neurotoxicity Research. 2022;**40**(2):670-686

[103] Lu G et al. Role and possible mechanisms of Sirt1 in depression. Oxidative Medicine and Cellular Longevity. 2018;**2018**:8596903

[104] Won E, Na KS, Kim YK. Associations between melatonin, neuroinflammation, and brain alterations in depression. International Journal of Molecular Sciences. 2021;**23**(1)

[105] Tonon AC et al. Melatonin and depression: A translational perspective from animal models to clinical studies. Frontiers in Psychiatry. 2021;**12**:638981

[106] Erdogan ME et al. The effects of lipoic acid on redox status in brain regions and systemic circulation in streptozotocin-induced sporadic Alzheimer's disease model. Metabolic Brain Disease. 2017;**32**(4):1017-1031

[107] Hung CW et al. Ageing and neurodegenerative diseases. Ageing Research Reviews. 2010;**9**(Suppl. 1):S36-S46

[108] Zhou L et al. Degeneration and energy shortage in the suprachiasmatic nucleus underlies the circadian rhythm disturbance in ApoE(−/−) mice: Implications for Alzheimer's disease. Scientific Reports. 2016;**6**:36335

[109] Cuesta S et al. Melatonin can improve insulin resistance and aging-induced pancreas alterations in senescence-accelerated prone male mice (SAMP8). Age (Dordrecht, Netherlands). 2013;**35**(3):659-671

[110] Cristofol R et al. Neurons from senescence-accelerated SAMP8 mice are protected against frailty by the sirtuin 1 promoting agents melatonin and resveratrol. Journal of Pineal Research. 2012;**52**(3):271-281

[111] Luo F et al. Melatonin and autophagy in aging-related neurodegenerative diseases. International Journal of Molecular Sciences. 2020;**21**(19)

[112] Chen D, Zhang T, Lee TH. Cellular mechanisms of melatonin: Insight from neurodegenerative diseases. Biomolecules. 2020;**10**(8)

[113] Wade AG et al. Add-on prolonged-release melatonin for cognitive function and sleep in mild to moderate Alzheimer's disease: A 6-month, randomized, placebo-controlled, multicenter trial. Clinical Interventions in Aging. 2014;**9**:947-961

[114] Singer C et al. A multicenter, placebo-controlled trial of melatonin for sleep disturbance in Alzheimer's disease. Sleep. 2003;**26**(7):893-901

[115] Riemersma-van der Lek RF et al. Effect of bright light and melatonin on cognitive and noncognitive function in elderly residents of group care facilities: A randomized controlled trial. JAMA. 2008;**299**(22):2642-2655

[116] Dowling GA et al. Melatonin and bright-light treatment for rest-activity disruption in institutionalized patients with Alzheimer's disease. Journal of the American Geriatrics Society. 2008;**56**(2):239-246

[117] Asayama K et al. Double blind study of melatonin effects on the sleep-wake rhythm, cognitive and non-cognitive functions in Alzheimer type dementia. Journal of Nippon Medical School. 2003;**70**(4):334-341

[118] Blum B et al. Melatonin in traumatic brain injury and cognition. Cureus. 2021;**13**(9):e17776

[119] Bell A et al. Traumatic brain injury, sleep, and melatonin-intrinsic changes with therapeutic potential. Clocks Sleep. 2023;**5**(2):177-203

[120] Zou P et al. Resveratrol pretreatment attenuates traumatic brain injury in rats by suppressing NLRP3 inflammasome activation via SIRT1. Molecular Medicine Reports. 2018;**17**(2):3212-3217

[121] Zhang YM et al. XingNaoJing injection ameliorates cerebral ischaemia/reperfusion injury via SIRT1-mediated inflammatory response inhibition. Pharmaceutical Biology. 2020;**58**(1):16-24

[122] Qu XY et al. XingNaoJing injections protect against cerebral ischemia/reperfusion injury and alleviate blood-brain barrier disruption in rats, through an underlying mechanism of NLRP3 inflammasomes suppression. Chinese Journal of Natural Medicines. 2019;**17**(7):498-505

[123] Xu X et al. Therapeutic effect of berberine on metabolic diseases: Both pharmacological data and clinical evidence. Biomedicine & Pharmacotherapy. 2021;**133**:110984

[124] Ungurianu A et al. Interleukins and redox impairment in type 2 diabetes mellitus: Mini-review and pilot study. Current Medical Research and Opinion. 2022;**38**(4):511-522

[125] Lu C et al. Novel role of the SIRT1 in endocrine and metabolic diseases. International Journal of Biological Sciences. 2023;**19**(2):484-501

[126] Gradinaru D et al. Insulin-leptin axis, cardiometabolic risk and oxidative stress in elderly with metabolic syndrome. Experimental and Clinical Endocrinology & Diabetes. 2018

[127] Jenwitheesuk A et al. Melatonin regulates aging and neurodegeneration through energy metabolism, epigenetics, autophagy and circadian rhythm pathways. International Journal of Molecular Sciences. 2014;**15**(9):16848-16884

[128] Gutierrez-Cuesta J et al. Evaluation of potential pro-survival pathways regulated by melatonin in a murine senescence model. Journal of Pineal Research. 2008;**45**(4):497-505

[129] Ostrowska Z et al. Influence of pinealectomy and long-term melatonin administration on GH-IGF-I axis function in male rats. Neuro Endocrinology Letters. 2001;**22**(4):255-262

[130] Tajes M et al. Anti-aging properties of melatonin in an in vitro murine senescence model: Involvement of the sirtuin 1 pathway. Journal of Pineal Research. 2009;**47**(3):228-237

[131] Vriend J, Sheppard MS, Borer KT. Melatonin increases serum growth hormone and insulin-like growth factor I (IGF-I) levels in male Syrian hamsters via hypothalamic neurotransmitters. Growth, Development, and Aging. 1990;**54**(4):165-171

[132] Wilking M et al. Circadian rhythm connections to oxidative stress: Implications for human health. Antioxidants & Redox Signaling. 2013;**19**(2):192-208

[133] Cai Y et al. Expression of clock genes Per1 and Bmal1 in total leukocytes in

health and Parkinson's disease. European Journal of Neurology. 2010;**17**(4):550-554

[134] Ding H et al. Decreased expression of Bmal2 in patients with Parkinson's disease. Neuroscience Letters. 2011;**499**(3):186-188

[135] Slats D et al. Reciprocal interactions between sleep, circadian rhythms and Alzheimer's disease: Focus on the role of hypocretin and melatonin. Ageing Research Reviews. 2013;**12**(1):188-200

[136] Almoosawi S et al. Chronotype: Implications for epidemiologic studies on chrono-nutrition and cardiometabolic health. Advances in Nutrition. 2019;**10**(1):30-42

[137] Cardinali DP, Hardeland R. Inflammaging, metabolic syndrome and melatonin: A call for treatment studies. Neuroendocrinology. 2017;**104**(4):382-397

[138] Purdel C, Ungurianu A, Margina D. Metabolic and metabolomic insights regarding the Omega-3 PUFAs intake in type 1 diabetes mellitus. Frontiers in Molecular Biosciences. 2021;**8**:783065

[139] Srinivasan V et al. Metabolic syndrome, its pathophysiology and the role of melatonin. Recent Patents on Endocrine Metabolic & Immune Drug Discovery. 2013;7(1):11-25

[140] Puchalski SS, Green JN, Rasmussen DD. Melatonin effect on rat body weight regulation in response to high-fat diet at middle age. Endocrine. 2003;**21**(2):163-167

[141] Wolden-Hanson T et al. Daily melatonin administration to middle-aged male rats suppresses body weight, intraabdominal adiposity, and plasma leptin and insulin independent of food intake and total body fat. Endocrinology. 2000;**141**(2):487-497

[142] Zanquetta MM et al. Calorie restriction reduces pinealectomy-induced insulin resistance by improving GLUT4 gene expression and its translocation to the plasma membrane. Journal of Pineal Research. 2003;**35**(3):141-148

[143] Nogueira TC et al. Absence of melatonin induces night-time hepatic insulin resistance and increased gluconeogenesis due to stimulation of nocturnal unfolded protein response. Endocrinology. 2011;**152**(4):1253-1263

[144] She M et al. NEU-P11, a novel melatonin agonist, inhibits weight gain and improves insulin sensitivity in high-fat/high-sucrose-fed rats. Pharmacological Research. 2009;**59**(4):248-253

[145] Karamitri A, Jockers R. Melatonin in type 2 diabetes mellitus and obesity. Nature Reviews. Endocrinology. 2019;**15**(2):105-125

[146] Sartori C et al. Melatonin improves glucose homeostasis and endothelial vascular function in high-fat diet-fed insulin-resistant mice. Endocrinology. 2009;**150**(12):5311-5317

[147] Tchio C et al. Removal of melatonin receptor type 1 signalling induces dyslipidaemia and hormonal changes in mice subjected to environmental circadian disruption. Endocrinology, Diabetes & Metabolism. 2021;**4**(1):e00171

[148] Jung KH et al. Melatonin downregulates nuclear erythroid 2-related factor 2 and nuclear factor-kappaB during prevention of oxidative liver injury in a dimethylnitrosamine model. Journal of Pineal Research. 2009;**47**(2):173-183

[149] Jung KH et al. Melatonin ameliorates cerulein-induced pancreatitis by

the modulation of nuclear erythroid 2-related factor 2 and nuclear factor-kappaB in rats. Journal of Pineal Research. 2010;**48**(3):239-250

[150] Peschke E. Melatonin, endocrine pancreas and diabetes. Journal of Pineal Research. 2008;**44**(1):26-40

[151] Peschke E et al. Melatonin and type 2 diabetes - a possible link? Journal of Pineal Research. 2007;**42**(4):350-358

[152] Huber M et al. Genetics of melatonin receptor type 2 is associated with left ventricular function in hypertensive patients treated according to guidelines. European Journal of Internal Medicine. 2013;**24**(7):650-655

[153] Prokopenko I et al. Variants in MTNR1B influence fasting glucose levels. Nature Genetics. 2009;**41**(1):77-81

[154] Zheng C et al. A common variant in the MTNR1b gene is associated with increased risk of impaired fasting glucose (IFG) in youth with obesity. Obesity (Silver Spring). 2015;**23**(5):1022-1029

[155] Gubin DG et al. Daily melatonin administration attenuates age-dependent disturbances of cardiovascular rhythms. Current Aging Science. 2016;**9**(1):5-13

[156] Tamura H et al. Melatonin treatment in peri- and postmenopausal women elevates serum high-density lipoprotein cholesterol levels without influencing total cholesterol levels. Journal of Pineal Research. 2008;**45**(1):101-105

[157] Gouspillou G et al. Protective role of parkin in skeletal muscle contractile and mitochondrial function. The Journal of Physiology. 2018;**596**(13):2565-2579

[158] Meynial-Denis D et al. New strategies to fight against sarcopenia at old age. Journal of Aging Research. 2012;**2012**:676042

[159] Stacchiotti A, Favero G, Rodella LF. Impact of melatonin on skeletal muscle and exercise. Cell. 2020;**9**(2)

[160] Salucci S et al. Melatonin role in skeletal muscle disorders. European Review for Medical and Pharmacological Sciences. 2021;**25**(2):1024-1033

[161] Pizzuto M, Pelegrin P. Cardiolipin in immune signaling and cell death. Trends in Cell Biology. 2020;**30**(11):892-903

[162] Li XX et al. Cardiolipin and its different properties in mitophagy and apoptosis. The Journal of Histochemistry and Cytochemistry. 2015;**63**(5):301-311

[163] Hibaoui Y et al. Melatonin improves muscle function of the dystrophic mdx5Cv mouse, a model for Duchenne muscular dystrophy. Journal of Pineal Research. 2011;**51**(2):163-171

[164] McCormick R, Vasilaki A. Age-related changes in skeletal muscle: Changes to life-style as a therapy. Biogerontology. 2018;**19**(6):519-536

[165] Heydemann A. Skeletal muscle metabolism in Duchenne and Becker muscular dystrophy-implications for therapies. Nutrients. 2018;**10**(6)

[166] Gomez-Pinilla PJ, Camello PJ, Pozo MJ. Protective effect of melatonin on Ca2+ homeostasis and contractility in acute cholecystitis. Journal of Pineal Research. 2008;**44**(3):250-260

[167] Yeung HM, Hung MW, Fung ML. Melatonin ameliorates calcium homeostasis in myocardial and ischemia-reperfusion injury in chronically hypoxic rats. Journal of Pineal Research. 2008;**45**(4):373-382

[168] Caumo W et al. Melatonin is a biomarker of circadian dysregulation and is correlated with major depression and fibromyalgia symptom severity. Journal of Pain Research. 2019;**12**:545-556

[169] Stratos I et al. Melatonin restores muscle regeneration and enhances muscle function after crush injury in rats. Journal of Pineal Research. 2012;**52**(1):62-70

[170] Cohen S. Role of calpains in promoting desmin filaments depolymerization and muscle atrophy. Biochimica et Biophysica Acta. 2020;**1867**(10):118788

[171] Smith IJ, Lecker SH, Hasselgren PO. Calpain activity and muscle wasting in sepsis. American Journal of Physiology. Endocrinology and Metabolism. 2008;**295**(4):E762-E771

[172] Tamtaji OR et al. Melatonin, a calpain inhibitor in the central nervous system: Current status and future perspectives. Journal of Cellular Physiology. 2019;**234**(2):1001-1007

[173] van den Beuken-van Everdingen MH et al. Update on prevalence of pain in patients with cancer: Systematic review and meta-analysis. Journal of Pain and Symptom Management. 2016;**51**(6):1070-1090 e9

[174] Talib WH. Melatonin and cancer hallmarks. Molecules. 2018;**23**(3)

[175] Reiter RJ et al. Melatonin, a full service anti-cancer agent: Inhibition of initiation, progression and metastasis. International Journal of Molecular Sciences. 2017;**18**(4)

[176] Reiter RJ et al. Light at night, chronodisruption, melatonin suppression, and cancer risk: A review. Critical Reviews in Oncogenesis. 2007;**13**(4):303-328

[177] Voiculescu SE et al. Behavioral and molecular effects of prenatal continuous light exposure in the adult rat. Brain Research. 2016;**1650**:51-59

[178] Blask DE et al. Melatonin-depleted blood from premenopausal women exposed to light at night stimulates growth of human breast cancer xenografts in nude rats. Cancer Research. 2005;**65**(23):11174-11184

[179] Jung-Hynes B et al. Melatonin, a novel Sirt1 inhibitor, imparts antiproliferative effects against prostate cancer in vitro in culture and in vivo in TRAMP model. Journal of Pineal Research. 2011;**50**(2):140-149

[180] Cheng Y et al. SIRT1 inhibition by melatonin exerts antitumor activity in human osteosarcoma cells. European Journal of Pharmacology. 2013;**715**(1-3):219-229

[181] Hill SM et al. Molecular mechanisms of melatonin anticancer effects. Integrative Cancer Therapies. 2009;**8**(4):337-346

[182] Proietti S et al. Melatonin down-regulates MDM2 gene expression and enhances p53 acetylation in MCF-7 cells. Journal of Pineal Research. 2014;**57**(1):120-129

[183] Frazzi R. SIRT1 in secretory organ cancer. Frontiers in Endocrinology (Lausanne). 2018;**9**:569

[184] Sharma A et al. Shedding light on structure, function and regulation of human sirtuins: A comprehensive review. 3 Biotech. 2023;**13**(1):29

[185] Rodriguez-Santana C et al. Role of melatonin in cancer: Effect on clock genes. International Journal of Molecular Sciences. 2023;**24**(3)

[186] Kritsilis M et al. Ageing, cellular senescence and neurodegenerative disease. International Journal of Molecular Sciences. 2018;**19**(10)

[187] Favero G et al. Melatonin: Protection against age-related cardiac pathology. Ageing Research Reviews. 2017;**35**:336-349

[188] Majidinia M et al. The role of melatonin, a multitasking molecule, in retarding the processes of ageing. Ageing Research Reviews. 2018;**47**:198-213

[189] Chang HC, Guarente L. SIRT1 mediates central circadian control in the SCN by a mechanism that decays with aging. Cell. 2013;**153**(7):1448-1460

[190] Franceschi C, Campisi J. Chronic inflammation (inflammaging) and its potential contribution to age-associated diseases. The Journals of Gerontology. Series A, Biological Sciences and Medical Sciences. 2014;**69**(Suppl. 1):S4-S9

[191] Kireev RA, Vara E, Tresguerres JA. Growth hormone and melatonin prevent age-related alteration in apoptosis processes in the dentate gyrus of male rats. Biogerontology. 2013;**14**(4):431-442

[192] Keskin-Aktan A et al. The effects of melatonin and curcumin on the expression of SIRT2, Bcl-2 and Bax in the hippocampus of adult rats. Brain Research Bulletin. 2018;**137**:306-310

[193] Keskin-Aktan A et al. SIRT2 and FOXO3a expressions in the cerebral cortex and hippocampus of young and aged male rats: Antioxidant and anti-apoptotic effects of melatonin. Biologia Futura. 2022;**73**(1):71-85

[194] Akbulut KG, Aktas SH, Akbulut H. The role of melatonin, sirtuin2 and FoXO1 transcription factor in the aging process of colon in male rats. Biogerontology. 2015;**16**(1):99-108

[195] Maestroni GJ et al. Does melatonin play a disease-promoting role in rheumatoid arthritis? Journal of Neuroimmunology. 2005;**158**(1-2):106-111

[196] Ghareghani M et al. Melatonin exacerbates acute experimental autoimmune encephalomyelitis by enhancing the serum levels of lactate: A potential biomarker of multiple sclerosis progression. Clinical and Experimental Pharmacology & Physiology. 2017;**44**(1):52-61

[197] Cutolo M, Maestroni GJ. The melatonin-cytokine connection in rheumatoid arthritis. Annals of the Rheumatic Diseases. 2005;**64**(8):1109-1111

[198] Spinedi E, Cardinali DP. Neuroendocrine-metabolic dysfunction and sleep disturbances in neurodegenerative disorders: Focus on Alzheimer's disease and melatonin. Neuroendocrinology. 2019;**108**(4):354-364

[199] Rosales-Corral SA et al. Alzheimer's disease: Pathological mechanisms and the beneficial role of melatonin. Journal of Pineal Research. 2012;**52**(2):167-202

Chapter 2

Aging Pathways: Unraveling Geriatric Neuropsychology and Innovative Neuromodulatory Treatments in the New Millennium

Chiara Di Fazio and Sara Palermo

Abstract

As the global population ages, distinguishing between the effects of chronic diseases and inherent aging challenges becomes paramount. The intersection of geriatric neuropsychology and gerontology provides a comprehensive framework to navigate these complexities. We will explore the foundational aspects of geriatric neuropsychology, surveying prominent theories of brain aging, structural and functional changes, and the intricate relationship between aging and neurodegenerative diseases. Acknowledging the relevance of frailty as a critical marker, the chapter emphasizes the importance of a comprehensive geriatric evaluation to guide nuanced interventions. A pivotal focus is then directed toward non-invasive neuromodulatory treatments, particularly transcranial magnetic stimulation (TMS), and its application in mitigating age-related cognitive decline. This exploration is contextualized within the broader framework of the medicine of complexity, recognizing the interconnectedness of various physiological and psychological factors in aging.

Keywords: ageotype, brain aging, comprehensive geriatric evaluation, neurogenesis, Hebbian plasticity, transcranial magnetic stimulation

1. Introduction

Aging, regardless of the specific age category it characterizes, should not be equated with a state of illness. Instead, it must be recognized as a natural phenomenon intricately linked with progressive physiological and psychological transformations in the organism. This aging process, marked by heightened biological vulnerability, can amplify the predisposition to various illnesses [1].

The process of aging is inherently diverse, with everyone undergoing a unique aging journey [2]. Aging is a gradual and continuous natural mutation involving the gradual decline of various bodily functions [2]. The life-span perspective recognizes functional changes as inherent to the human aging process, distinguishing between pure aging and its continuum toward pathological aging [3, 4].

Distinct aging patterns, or ageotypes, have been identified based on molecular pathway changes over time, including metabolic, immune, hepatic, and nephrotic ageotypes [5]. This molecular classification provides a personalized assessment of aging, reflects lifestyle and medical history, and offers insights into potential health risk factors.

Multimorbidity and polypharmacotherapy weaken the body, predisposing individuals to accelerated aging and frailty, which is considered the most challenging expression of aging [1, 2]. Frailty is an integrated and multidimensional condition where biological, functional, psychological, and social factors interact, posing risks for deteriorating mental health and cognitive decline [6–9]. Cognitive frailty specifically refers to the co-occurrence of mild cognitive impairment and physical frailty without a major neurocognitive disorder diagnosis [10].

1.1 The imperative of distinguishing effects: Chronic diseases vs. aging challenges

The biological process of aging is characterized by a complex interplay of molecular, cellular, and systemic changes, encompassing alterations in genetic expression, cellular functions, and tissue integrity. These changes occur gradually over time, leading to a progressive transformation of both physiological and psychological dimensions. On a molecular level, aging involves intricate mechanisms such as telomere shortening, genomic instability, and mitochondrial dysfunction, contributing to cellular senescence and ultimately influencing the entire organism [11].

Crucially, it is imperative to emphasize that aging, in its essence, is not synonymous with a pathological state. Aging should be conceptualized as a dynamic, natural phenomenon that reflects the intricate orchestration of biological processes over the lifespan of an organism. The complexity arises from the fact that aging and chronic diseases, prevalent in the elderly population, share commonalities in their manifestations. This includes physiological declines, such as decreased organ function and immune system efficacy, which can be attributed to both aging and the development of chronic conditions [12, 13].

The challenge lies in discerning between age-related changes and those induced by specific chronic diseases, given their propensity to exhibit overlapping clinical characteristics. For instance, cognitive decline, a common feature of aging, can also manifest in neurodegenerative conditions like Alzheimer's disease. Distinguishing these nuances is crucial for accurate diagnosis and tailored interventions.

The field of geriatric neuropsychology plays a pivotal role in unraveling these complexities. It involves in-depth assessments of cognitive functions, neurobiological markers, and psychosocial factors to differentiate between age-related cognitive changes and pathological conditions [14]. Advanced imaging techniques, such as functional magnetic resonance imaging (fMRI) and positron emission tomography (PET), provide insights into the structural and functional alterations occurring in the aging brain, aiding in the identification of age-related patterns versus disease-related changes [15, 16].

1.2 The intersect of geriatric neuropsychology and gerontology

Geriatric neuropsychology and gerontology represent two interdisciplinary fields that converge to provide a comprehensive understanding of the complexities associated with aging. Gerontology, as a broader discipline, explores aging from a holistic perspective, considering the social, cultural, psychological, intellectual, and biological aspects of the aging process [17–19].

In the realm of gerontology, the focus extends beyond the individual to encompass the societal implications of an aging population. The interdisciplinary nature of gerontology integrates insights from sociology, anthropology, and public health to examine the impact of aging on communities, healthcare systems, and societal structures. This perspective is crucial for addressing the challenges and opportunities presented by an aging demographic on a global scale.

Geriatric neuropsychology, on the other hand, zooms in on the intricate relationship between aging and the brain. It investigates how the physiological changes associated with aging affect cognitive functions, emotional well-being, and overall mental health. This field employs a range of specialized assessments, including cognitive tests, neuroimaging, and psychosocial evaluations, to unravel the complexities of age-related changes in the brain [18].

The intersection of geriatric neuropsychology and gerontology is where these two disciplines harmonize, creating a synergistic approach to understanding the multifaceted aspects of aging. Geriatric neuropsychology contributes valuable insights into the cognitive and neurological dimensions of aging, shedding light on how changes in the brain impact an individual's overall well-being.

For instance, in studying cognitive aging, geriatric neuropsychologists explore how age-related changes in brain structure and function may manifest in cognitive decline, memory impairment, or other neuropsychological conditions. This information is then integrated into the broader gerontological framework, enabling a more comprehensive understanding of how cognitive health influences an individual's ability to engage with their social environment and maintain autonomy in daily activities.

The cooperation between geriatric neuropsychology and gerontology is vital in customizing interventions to meet the distinct requirements of the aging demographic. By amalgamating insights from these two fields, researchers and practitioners can formulate comprehensive approaches aimed at fostering cognitive health, emotional well-being, and the overall quality of life for older individuals. This convergence serves as a pivotal junction, propelling the progression of our understanding and elevating the standard of care.

2. Foundational aspects of geriatric neuropsychology

In delving into the intricate domain of geriatric neuropsychology, it becomes imperative to unravel the foundational aspects that underpin our understanding of the dynamic interplay between aging and the intricate workings of the human brain. This inquiry guides us toward the fundamental principles and theories that elucidate the intricate terrain where neurological processes intersect with the challenges presented by the process of advancing age.

2.1 Surveying prominent theories of "brain aging"

Brain aging encompasses a complex array of molecular and structural changes that collectively influence cognitive function and neurological well-being. Contemporary research has significantly advanced our comprehension of these intricacies, shedding light on tangible alterations observed in the aging brain [20, 21].

At its core, brain aging involves a gradual decline in cognitive abilities and neurological functions. Genetic predispositions and environmental factors intricately interact, shaping an individual's susceptibility to age-related neurodegeneration. Molecular mechanisms such as telomere shortening, increased oxidative stress, and chronic neuroinflammation have emerged as pivotal contributors to cellular senescence and diminished neural plasticity, hallmarking the aging brain [22, 23].

Cutting-edge neuroimaging technologies have played a pivotal role in discerning the structural and functional modifications occurring in the aging brain. fMRI and PET have enabled the observation of connectivity patterns, alterations in synaptic integrity, and changes in regional brain activity. These tools provide tangible evidence of age-related neural degeneration, allowing researchers to correlate cognitive decline with specific anatomical and functional variations [24]. Concrete changes observed in brain aging include atrophy in certain brain regions, particularly the hippocampus and prefrontal cortex, areas crucial for memory and executive functions [25, 26]. Additionally, altered patterns of neurotransmitter activity, diminished synaptic density, and the presence of beta-amyloid plaques are indicative of age-related cognitive decline, often associated with conditions like Alzheimer's disease [27].

Our contemporary understanding of brain aging is marked by a detailed exploration of molecular processes, structural modifications, and observable changes in neural functioning. This nuanced approach not only refines our grasp of cognitive aging but also holds promise for developing targeted interventions to mitigate age-related cognitive decline and enhance the overall neurological health of the aging population. One of the key findings pertains to the concept of *brain reserve*, which refers to the brain's inherent ability to withstand and compensate for age-related changes or pathological conditions without exhibiting noticeable cognitive decline [28, 29]. Another key concept is that of *cognitive reserve*, where individuals with enriched cognitive experiences exhibit greater resilience against age-related cognitive decline (see **Table 1**) [28, 30].

Importantly, continuous intellectual engagement and cognitive stimulation throughout life contribute to enhanced neuroplasticity, acting as a protective factor against the impact of aging on cognitive functions.

2.2 Structural and functional changes in the aging brain

The aging process entails a nuanced interplay of structural and functional modifications within the brain, influencing its overall cognitive architecture. Delving into these changes provides a comprehensive understanding of the intricacies associated with aging-related cognitive variations.

2.2.1 Structural alterations

- *Gray matter decline*: Aging is marked by a discernible reduction in gray matter volume, particularly pronounced in regions crucial for memory and cognitive functions. The hippocampus, integral to memory formation, and the prefrontal cortex, responsible for executive functions, are notably affected [31, 32]. These structural changes may contribute to the observed decline in specific cognitive abilities.

- *White matter integrity and connectivity*: Concurrently, alterations in white matter integrity and connectivity patterns occur. The white matter, consisting of nerve fibers, experiences changes that impact the speed at which information is

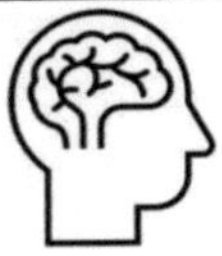 **Brain reserve**	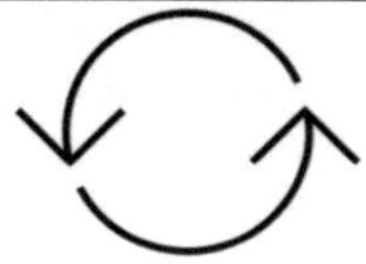	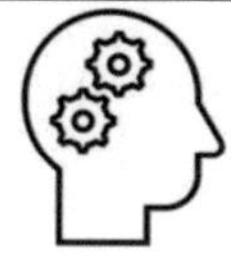 **Cognitive reserve**
Brain reserve refers to the brain's inherent ability to withstand and compensate for age-related changes or pathological conditions without exhibiting noticeable cognitive decline.	Definition	Cognitive reserve is the mind's ability to maintain optimal cognitive functioning and resilience against age-related changes or neurological damage.
It involves the structural and functional resilience of the brain, enabling the maintenance of cognitive function in the presence of damage or degeneration.	Components	It involves the dynamic interplay between lifelong cognitive experiences, intellectual pursuits, and neural adaptability.
Brain reserve is influenced by various factors, including genetic predispositions, neural plasticity, and the efficiency of neural networks.	Influence	Cognitive reserve significantly influences an individual's capacity to withstand cognitive decline or neurological disorders.
The brain's robust structural and functional resilience enables the preservation of cognitive function, even when confronted with damage or degeneration. This resilience is particularly notable in the intricate network of brain connections, known as functional connectome, and is exemplified by the brain's ability to operate effectively in a resting state, sustaining essential cognitive functions despite potential structural challenges.	Manifestation	Individuals with a history of mentally stimulating activities and diverse cognitive engagements are likely to exhibit a greater ability to cope with and compensate for the effects of aging or neurological challenges.
Individuals with a higher brain reserve may experience a delay in the onset of cognitive symptoms or a slower progression of cognitive decline in the face of aging or neurological diseases.	Outcome	The preservation of cognitive abilities and the promotion of overall brain health are key outcomes associated with a higher cognitive reserve.
Engaging in intellectually stimulating activities and maintaining a cognitively enriching lifestyle are believed to contribute to the development and enhancement of brain reserve over the lifespan.	Contributing factors	Cognitive reserve is shaped by a myriad of factors, including the extent of lifelong cognitive engagement, educational background, occupational complexity, and socio-intellectual activities. Furthermore, genetic predispositions, cultural exposures, and the quality of interpersonal relationships contribute significantly to the development and enhancement of cognitive reserve throughout an individual's lifespan.

Table 1.
Key aspects of cognitive and brain reserve: Understanding the capacities and influences that contribute to maintaining optimal cognitive functioning and resilience, as well as the brain's inherent ability to withstand age-related changes or pathological conditions, with associated contributing factors and outcomes.

processed across different brain regions. Disruptions in white matter connectivity can influence the efficiency of communication between brain areas, affecting cognitive processing [33, 34].

2.2.2 Functional shifts

- *Neural activity dynamics*: Functionally, the aging brain undergoes shifts in neural activity. Various studies report both increases and decreases in activity within different brain regions during different cognitive tasks. These fluctuations may reflect adaptive responses or compensatory mechanisms as the brain adjusts to aging-related changes [35–37].

- *Neurotransmitter decline*: Accompanying these shifts is a decline in neurotransmitter activity, crucial for transmitting signals between neurons. Neurotransmitters like dopamine, serotonin, and acetylcholine play vital roles in cognitive functions such as attention, memory, and mood regulation. Their reduction can impact inter-neuronal communication and contribute to cognitive variability [21, 38, 39].

Understanding these intricate structural and functional changes is pivotal for developing targeted interventions aimed at preserving cognitive abilities in older individuals. Ongoing research endeavors strive to unravel the complexities of the aging brain, fostering innovative strategies to enhance cognitive well-being and quality of life in the elderly.

2.3 Intricate relationship between aging and neurodegenerative diseases

The intricate relationship between aging and neurodegenerative diseases unveils a complex interplay of biological processes that significantly impact the trajectory of cognitive health in older individuals. Aging itself is accompanied by structural and functional changes in the brain, as seen in the decline of gray matter volume and alterations in neural activity. Neurodegenerative diseases, on the other hand, represent a distinct category of disorders marked by the progressive degeneration of specific neural structures, leading to cognitive decline. While aging is a natural and universal process, the risk of neurodegenerative diseases increases with age. Conditions such as Alzheimer's and Parkinson's diseases exemplify the convergence of aging-related changes and pathological processes, resulting in exacerbated cognitive impairment. Understanding this intricate relationship is crucial for developing comprehensive approaches to support cognitive well-being in the elderly and to differentiate age-related cognitive changes from those associated with neurodegenerative disorders, allowing for timely interventions and improved quality of life.

2.4 Brain reserve and cognitive reserve: Buffering cognitive decline

Brain reserve and cognitive reserve play crucial roles in mitigating cognitive decline as individuals age. Brain reserve, indicative of the brain's inherent robustness, empowers it to endure age-related changes or pathological conditions without displaying noticeable cognitive impairment [28, 29]. Meanwhile, cognitive reserve involves the mind's ability to sustain optimal cognitive functioning by actively participating in intellectually stimulating activities and diverse cognitive experiences throughout one's life [28, 30]. These reserves act as protective mechanisms, allowing individuals to effectively manage and compensate for the cognitive effects of aging. Engaging in continuous learning, pursuing intellectually challenging tasks, and maintaining social and cognitive activities contribute significantly to the fortification of cognitive reserve. A comprehensive understanding of the functions of the brain and cognitive reserve provides valuable insights for developing strategies aimed at promoting cognitive health, delaying cognitive decline, and ultimately enhancing the overall quality of life for aging individuals.

Imagine an individual who, throughout their life, consistently engaged in mentally challenging activities, pursued diverse learning experiences, and maintained a socially active lifestyle. This person, with a well-developed cognitive reserve, possesses a greater capacity to navigate the challenges of aging without experiencing a pronounced decline in cognitive functions. The brain reserve, acting as a robust shield, enables this individual to withstand age-related structural and functional changes without significant cognitive impairment. This example underscores the practical implications of actively fostering brain and cognitive reserve. By incorporating intellectually stimulating activities into their daily lives, individuals can potentially delay the onset of cognitive decline and sustain a higher level of cognitive functioning in later years. The buffering effect provided by these reserves offers a tangible pathway toward promoting cognitive health and enhancing the overall well-being of aging individuals.

3. Relevance of frailty as a critical marker

Frailty stands as a pivotal marker in the aging process, representing a state of heightened vulnerability to negative health outcomes due to a reduction in functional reserves across multiple organ systems [40–42]. Its significance extends beyond physical aspects, influencing various dimensions of an individual's well-being, including cognitive health.

Frailty is not merely a consequence of aging but rather a comprehensive reflection of an individual's physiological and psychological state. It encapsulates the dynamic interplay between biological, cognitive, and socio-economic factors, making it a valuable marker for assessing the overall health status of an aging individual [43, 44]. Understanding frailty provides insights into the complexities of the aging process, allowing for targeted interventions that address the multifaceted needs of older adults.

Frailty, as a critical marker in the aging process, plays a substantial role in influencing cognitive decline, with scientific evidence highlighting its intricate association with neurocognitive outcomes. Numerous studies have demonstrated a clear link between frailty and an increased risk of cognitive impairment and neurocognitive disorders in the elderly [45, 46].

Research by Robertson and colleagues [47] found that frail individuals exhibit a higher likelihood of developing mild cognitive impairment (MCI) compared to their non-frail counterparts. The study, spanning a longitudinal analysis of aging cohorts, revealed that the presence of frailty significantly accelerated the progression from MCI to more severe cognitive impairments, such as Alzheimer's disease and related dementias.

Moreover, a comprehensive meta-analysis conducted by Panza et al. [48] emphasized the role of frailty as a predictor of an incident major neurocognitive disorder. The review encompassed diverse population-based studies, consistently establishing frailty as an independent risk factor for the onset of major neurocognitive disorders. The mechanisms underlying this association involve a complex interplay of vascular, inflammatory, and neurodegenerative processes, amplifying the impact of frailty on cognitive trajectories [48].

Understanding the intricate relationship between frailty and cognitive decline not only provides valuable prognostic insights but also opens avenues for targeted interventions. Interventions aimed at mitigating frailty, such as personalized exercise programs and nutritional interventions, have shown promise in preserving cognitive function and slowing down the progression of cognitive decline in frail individuals [49, 50]. In addition, today's developments pave the way for non-invasive neuromodulatory treatments capable of enhancing brain reserve or mitigating potential pathological outcomes through neuromodulation interventions. Recognizing frailty as a crucial determinant of cognitive health underscores the importance of comprehensive geriatric assessments and interventions to enhance the overall well-being of older adults.

4. Comprehensive geriatric evaluation: guiding nuanced interventions

Comprehensive geriatric evaluation stands as a cornerstone in tailoring nuanced interventions for the aging population, addressing the multifaceted aspects of health in older individuals. The significance of comprehensive geriatric evaluation lies in its ability to provide a thorough understanding of an elderly individual's health status, encompassing physical, cognitive, and socio-economic dimensions [51, 52]. This holistic assessment involves a multidisciplinary approach, integrating medical, psychological, and functional evaluations [53]. Components may include detailed medical histories, functional assessments, cognitive screenings, and social support evaluations, ensuring a comprehensive grasp of an individual's unique needs [54].

Within the framework of evaluation, addressing frailty emerges as a crucial component. Identifying frailty allows for targeted interventions that consider an individual's vulnerability and tailor care plans accordingly. Frailty assessments often involve evaluating physical strength, mobility, nutrition, and psychosocial factors, providing a comprehensive understanding of an individual's overall health and potential areas of intervention. This comprehensive evaluation not only informs personalized care plans but also sets the stage for exploring innovative interventions, including non-invasive neuromodulatory treatments.

The subsequent paragraph will delve into the promising realm of non-invasive neuromodulation as a potential avenue for enhancing cognitive well-being within the geriatric population.

5. Non-invasive neuromodulatory treatments

Non-invasive neuromodulation is an advanced field that targets brain activity to induce changes in behavioral or motor-sensory functions without necessitating invasive procedures [54]. This methodology encompasses various techniques, including transcranial direct current stimulation (tDCS) or alternating current stimulation (tACS), characterized by small, painless electrical discharges, and transcranial magnetic stimulation (TMS), which employs electromagnetic waves. The primary distinction among these methodologies lies in the equipment used and the depth of action. tDCS involves the application of low-level, constant electrical current to the brain *via* electrodes placed on the scalp, which is known for its painless nature and its ability to modulate neuronal activity, making it a promising tool for various applications in cognitive enhancement, motor rehabilitation, and psychiatric disorders [55], while tACS delivers rhythmic electrical stimulation to the brain at specific frequencies. This method has shown potential in modulating neural oscillations and has been investigated for its role in enhancing cognitive functions, such as memory and attention, as well as for its therapeutic potential in neurological and psychiatric conditions [56]. TMS, on the contrary, is a non-invasive stimulation technique that employs electromagnetic waves to stimulate specific brain regions [57].

Indeed, all these methodologies derive their proven efficacy from the concept of *neuroplasticity.* According to this hypothesis, numerous nervous system disorders stem from an imbalance between stressors (which target specific structures based on individual vulnerability rooted in genetic predisposition) and neuroplasticity factors (the central nervous system's ability to generate new cells and connections) [58]. Physical, magnetic, light, and electrostatic stimuli function by activating the structures involved in *neurogenesis* [59, 60]. The stimulation those techniques provide is aligned with the principles of Hebbian plasticity, where repeated activation of neuronal pathways strengthens synaptic connections [58]. This phenomenon, known as Hebbian learning, underscores the adaptability of the nervous system in response to stimuli [61]. Consequently, the application of neuromodulation techniques harnesses the principles of Hebbian plasticity to promote neurogenesis, aiming to counteract the detrimental effects of stressors and foster a resilient nervous system [62].

5.1 Transcranial magnetic stimulation (TMS): mitigating age-related cognitive decline

TMS emerges as a leading non-invasive neuromodulatory technique, demonstrating efficacy in modulating neural activity and potentially ameliorating cognitive decline associated with aging [63, 64]. TMS is a non-invasive neuromodulatory technique that involves the application of rapidly changing magnetic fields to specific brain regions. This process induces electrical currents in the targeted areas of the brain, leading to the depolarization or hyperpolarization of neurons. By modulating neuronal activity, TMS has been shown to promote neuroplasticity [57] and influence neuronal connectivity. Research suggests its potential to enhance cognitive functions, making it a compelling intervention in the quest to preserve cognitive health in older individuals [63]. Exploring case studies and empirical evidence further bolsters the case for TMS in geriatric neuropsychology. Investigations into the application of TMS to older adults reveal promising outcomes, including improvements in memory, attention, and executive functions. The non-invasiveness of TMS, coupled with its relatively low side effect profile, enhances its appeal as a viable option for age-related cognitive challenges. Unlike invasive procedures, TMS does not require surgery or anesthesia, and it is generally well-tolerated by individuals. This makes it an attractive option for older adults, who may be more vulnerable to the risks associated with invasive interventions. As non-invasive neuromodulation continues to advance, TMS stands out as a beacon of hope in the endeavor to tailor interventions that promote cognitive health, independence, and an enriched quality of life for the elderly. The exploration of TMS efficacy in geriatric neuropsychology underscores the evolving landscape of innovative treatments dedicated to addressing the unique needs of an aging population, offering new possibilities for enhancing cognitive function and overall well-being in older individuals.

6. Conclusions

Aging unfolds as a complex interplay of physiological changes, rendering the elderly more susceptible to various health challenges. Thus, within the realm of geriatric neuropsychology, the need to discern between the distinct trajectories of aging and chronic diseases becomes paramount. This imperative recognition lays the foundation for developing targeted interventions, acknowledging the nuanced intricacies of the aging process, and enabling a more personalized and effective approach to geriatric care. The synergistic collaboration between geriatric neuropsychology and gerontology emerges as a fundamental reference point for shaping interventions tailored to the unique needs of the aging population. By integrating perspectives from both disciplines, researchers and practitioners can develop holistic strategies that not only promote cognitive health, emotional well-being, and overall quality of life for older individuals but also leverage innovative approaches such as transcranial magnetic stimulation (TMS) and Hebbian plasticity. This union represents a crucial nexus, catalyzing the advancement of our knowledge and enhancing the care and support provided to the elderly in the continually evolving landscape of the twenty-first century.

Acknowledgements

No funding was available to the authors.

Conflict of interest

The authors declare that the manuscript was written in the absence of any commercial or financial relationships that could be construed as a potential conflict of interest.

Author details

Chiara Di Fazio[1,2] and Sara Palermo[1,3]*

1 Department of Psychology, University of Turin, Turin, Italy

2 International School of Advanced Studies, University of Camerino, Camerino, Italy

3 Neuroradiology Unit, Department of Diagnostic and Technology, Fondazione IRCCS Istituto Neurologico Carlo Besta, Milan, Italy

*Address all correspondence to: sara.palermo@unito.it

References

[1] Morese R, Palermo S, Defedele M, Nervo J, Borraccino A. Vulnerability and social exclusion: Risk in adolescence and old age. In: Morese R, Palermo S, editors. The New Forms of Social Exclusion. London: IntechOpen Limited; 2019. pp. 1-16. DOI: 10.5772/intechopen.85463

[2] Palermo S. Covid-19 Pandemic: Maximizing future vaccination treatments considering aging and frailty. Frontiers in Medicine. 2020;7:558835. DOI: 10.3389/fmed.2020.558835

[3] Smith GE, Bondi MW. Mild Cognitive Impairment and Dementia: Definitions, Diagnosis, and Treatment. Oxford: OUP USA; 2013. 416 p. ISBN: 0199764182

[4] Wise DA. Analyses in the Economics of Aging. Chicago: University of Chicago Press; 2005. 416 p. ISBN: 0-226-90286-2

[5] Ahadi S, Zhou W, Schüssler-Fiorenza Rose SM, et al. Personal aging markers and ageotypes revealed by deep longitudinal profiling. Nature Medicine. 2020;**26**(1):83-90. DOI: 10.1038/s41591-019-0719-5

[6] Gobbens RJ, Luijkx KG, Wijnen-Sponselee MT, Schols JM. In search of an integral conceptual definition of frailty: Opinions of experts. Journal of the American Medical Directors Association. 2010;**11**(5):338-343. DOI: 10.1016/j.jamda.2009.09.015

[7] Sourial N, Wolfson C, Bergman H, et al. A correspondence analysis revealed frailty deficits aggregate and are multidimensional. Journal of Clinical Epidemiology. 2010;**63**(6):647-654. DOI: 10.1016/j.jclinepi.2009.08.007

[8] Ní Mhaoláin AM, Fan CW, Romero-Ortuno R, et al. Frailty, depression, and anxiety in later life. International Psychogeriatrics. 2012;**24**(8):1265-1274. DOI: 10.1017/S1041610211002110

[9] Nishiguchi S, Yamada M, Fukutani N, et al. Differential association of frailty with cognitive decline and sarcopenia in community-dwelling older adults. Journal of the American Medical Directors Association. 2015;**16**(2):120-124. DOI: 10.1016/j.jamda.2014.07.010

[10] Kelaiditi E, Cesari M, Canevelli M, et al. Cognitive frailty: Rational and definition from an (I.A.N.A./I.A.G.G.) international consensus group. The Journal of Nutrition, Health & Aging. 2013;**17**(9):726-734. DOI: 10.1007/s12603-013-0367-2

[11] da Costa JP, Vitorino R, Silva GM, Vogel C, Duarte AC, Rocha-Santos T. A synopsis on aging-theories, mechanisms and future prospects. Ageing Research Reviews. 2016;**29**:90-112. DOI: 10.1016/j.arr.2016.06.005

[12] Gilbert SF. Developmental biology. In: Aging: The Biology of Senescence. 6th ed. Sunderland (MA): Sinauer Associates; 2000. Available from: https://www.ncbi.nlm.nih.gov/books/NBK10041/

[13] Voropai D, Kroeskop A. Catching the aging curve early. Journal of Cosmetic Dermatology. 2023;**22**(Suppl. 1):28-31. DOI: 10.1111/jocd.15701

[14] Lu PH, Lee GJ. The role of neuropsychology in the assessment of the cognitively impaired elderly. Neurologic Clinics. 2017;**35**(2):191-206. DOI: 10.1016/j.ncl.2017.01.002

[15] Cole JH. Multimodality neuroimaging brain-age in UK biobank:

Relationship to biomedical, lifestyle, and cognitive factors. Neurobiology of Aging. 2020;**92**:34-42. DOI: 10.1016/j.neurobiolaging.2020.03.014

[16] Bethlehem RAI, Seidlitz J, White SR, et al. Brain charts for the human lifespan [published correction appears in nature. 2022 Oct;610(7931):E6]. Nature. 2022;**604**(7906):525-533. DOI: 10.1038/s41586-022-04554-y

[17] Schneider EL. The aging of the aged: Challenges for gerontology & geriatrics in the United States. Nihon Ronen Igakkai zasshi. Japanese journal of Geriatrics. 1992;**29**(4):245-247. DOI: 10.3143/geriatrics.29.245

[18] Smith AM. Geriatric neuropsychology: Assessment and intervention edited by Deborah K. Attix Kathleen A. Welsh-Bohmer. Educational Gerontology. 2007;**34**(1):101-102. DOI: 10.1080/03601270701764058

[19] Martin TA, Bush SS. Ethical considerations in geriatric neuropsychology. NeuroRehabilitation. 2008;**23**(5):447-454

[20] Peters R. Ageing and the brain. Postgraduate Medical Journal. 2006;**82**(964):84-88. DOI: 10.1136/pgmj.2005.036665

[21] Lee J, Kim HJ. Normal aging induces changes in the brain and neurodegeneration progress: Review of the structural, biochemical, metabolic, cellular, and molecular changes. Frontiers in Aging Neuroscience. 2022;**14**:931536. DOI: 10.3389/fnagi.2022.931536

[22] Wyss-Coray T. Ageing, neurodegeneration and brain rejuvenation. Nature. 2016;**539**(7628):180-186. DOI: 10.1038/nature20411

[23] Azam S, Haque ME, Balakrishnan R, Kim IS, Choi DK. The ageing brain: Molecular and cellular basis of neurodegeneration. Frontiers in Cell and Development Biology. 2021;**9**:683459. DOI: 10.3389/fcell.2021.683459

[24] Bigos KL, Hariri AR. Neuroimaging: Technologies at the interface of genes, brain, and behavior. Neuroimaging Clinics of North America. 2007;**17**(4):459-467, viii. DOI: 10.1016/j.nic.2007.09.005

[25] Jellinger KA, Attems J. Neuropathological approaches to cerebral aging and neuroplasticity. Dialogues in Clinical Neuroscience. 2013;**15**(1):29-43. DOI: 10.31887/DCNS.2013.15.1/kjellinger

[26] Toepper M. Dissociating normal aging from Alzheimer's disease: A view from cognitive neuroscience. Journal of Alzheimer's Disease. 2017;**57**(2):331-352. DOI: 10.3233/JAD-161099

[27] DeTure MA, Dickson DW. The neuropathological diagnosis of Alzheimer's disease. Molecular Neurodegeneration. 2019;**14**(1):32. DOI: 10.1186/s13024-019-0333-5

[28] Stern Y, Barnes CA, Grady C, Jones RN, Raz N. Brain reserve, cognitive reserve, compensation, and maintenance: Operationalization, validity, and mechanisms of cognitive resilience. Neurobiology of Aging. 2019;**83**:124-129. DOI: 10.1016/j.neurobiolaging.2019.03.022

[29] Hachinski V, Avan A. A new definition of brain reserve. Alzheimer's & Dementia. 2022;**18**(3):535-537. DOI: 10.1002/alz.12562

[30] Stern Y. Cognitive reserve in ageing and Alzheimer's disease. Lancet Neurology. 2012;**11**(11):1006-1012. DOI: 10.1016/S1474-4422(12)70191-6

[31] Terribilli D, Schaufelberger MS, Duran FL, et al. Age-related gray matter volume changes in the brain during non-elderly adulthood. Neurobiology of Aging. 2011;**32**(2):354-368. DOI: 10.1016/j.neurobiolaging. 2009.02.008

[32] Morrison JH, Baxter MG. The ageing cortical synapse: Hallmarks and implications for cognitive decline. Nature Reviews. Neuroscience. 2012;**13**(4):240-250. DOI: 10.1038/nrn3200

[33] Samson RD, Barnes CA. Impact of aging brain circuits on cognition. The European Journal of Neuroscience. 2013;**37**(12):1903-1915. DOI: 10.1111/ejn.12183

[34] Yang AC, Tsai SJ, Liu ME, Huang CC, Lin CP. The association of aging with white matter integrity and functional connectivity hubs. Frontiers in Aging Neuroscience. 2016;**8**:143. DOI: 10.3389/fnagi.2016.00143

[35] Andrews-Hanna JR, Snyder AZ, Vincent JL, Lustig C, Head D, Raichle ME, et al. Disruption of large-scale brain systems in advanced aging. Neuron. 2007;**56**(5):924-935. DOI: 10.1016/j.neuron.2007.10.038

[36] McDonough IM, Nolin SA, Visscher KM. 25 years of neurocognitive aging theories: What have we learned? Frontiers in Aging Neuroscience. 2022;**14**:1002096. DOI: 10.3389/fnagi.2022.1002096

[37] Dimitriadis SI, Castells-Sánchez A, Roig-Coll F, et al. Intrinsic functional brain connectivity changes following aerobic exercise, computerized cognitive training, and their combination in physically inactive healthy late-middle-aged adults: The Projecte Moviment. Geroscience. 2024;**46**(1):573-596. DOI: 10.1007/s11357-023-00946-8

[38] Teleanu RI, Niculescu AG, Roza E, Vladâcenco O, Grumezescu AM, Teleanu DM. Neurotransmitters-key factors in neurological and neurodegenerative disorders of the central nervous system. International Journal of Molecular Sciences. 2022;**23**(11):5954. DOI: 10.3390/ijms23115954

[39] Chen Y, Xu J, Chen Y. Regulation of neurotransmitters by the gut microbiota and effects on cognition in neurological disorders. Nutrients. 2021;**13**(6):2099. DOI: 10.3390/nu13062099 [Accessed: Jun 19, 2021]

[40] Xue QL. The frailty syndrome: Definition and natural history. Clinics in Geriatric Medicine. 2011;**27**(1):1-15. DOI: 10.1016/j.cger.2010.08.009

[41] Clegg A, Young J. The frailty syndrome. Clinical Medicine (London, England). 2011;**11**(1):72-75. DOI: 10.7861/clinmedicine.11-1-72

[42] Lozupone M, Solfrizzi V, Sardone R, et al. The epigenetics of frailty. Epigenomics. 2024;**16**(3):189-202. DOI: 10.2217/epi-2023-0279

[43] Pinheiro IM, de Aguiar DS, Dos Santos DM, de Jesus MBDC, da Silva FM, Costa DF, et al. Biopsychosocial factors associated with the frailty and pre-frailty among older adults. Geriatric Nursing. 2019;**40**(6):597-602. DOI: 10.1016/j.gerinurse.2019.06.002

[44] Polidori MC, Ferrucci L. Frailty from conceptualization to action: The biopsychosocial model of frailty and resilience. Aging Clinical and Experimental Research. 2023;**35**(4):725-727. DOI: 10.1007/s40520-022-02337-z

[45] Borges MK, Canevelli M, Cesari M, Aprahamian I. Frailty as a predictor of cognitive disorders: A systematic review and meta-analysis. Frontiers in Medicine

(Lausanne). 2019;**6**:26. DOI: 10.3389/fmed.2019.00026

[46] Li C, Ge S, Yin Y, Tian C, Mei Y, Han P. Frailty is associated with worse cognitive functioning in older adults. Frontiers in Psychiatry. 2023;**14**:1108902. DOI: 10.3389/fpsyt.2023.1108902

[47] Robertson DA, Savva GM, Kenny RA. Frailty and cognitive impairment–A review of the evidence and causal mechanisms. Ageing Research Reviews. 2013;**12**(4):840-851. DOI: 10.1016/j.arr.2013.06.004

[48] Panza F, Lozupone M, Solfrizzi V, Sardone R, Dibello V, Di Lena L, et al. Different cognitive frailty models and health- and cognitive-related outcomes in older age: From epidemiology to prevention. Journal of Alzheimer's Disease. 2018;**62**(3):993-1012. DOI: 10.3233/JAD-170963

[49] Kojima G, Iliffe S, Jivraj S, Walters K. Association between frailty and quality of life among community-dwelling older people: A systematic review and meta-analysis. Journal of Epidemiology and Community Health. 2016;**70**(7):716-721. DOI: 10.1136/jech-2015-206717

[50] Soll-Morka A, Kurpas D. The degree of meeting the needs of older people with frailty syndrome in the residential environment in relation to interventions-experimental study. International Journal of Environmental Research and Public Health. 2022;**19**(18):11682. DOI: 10.3390/ijerph191811682

[51] Devons CA. Comprehensive geriatric assessment: Making the most of the aging years. Current Opinion in Clinical Nutrition and Metabolic Care. 2002;**5**(1):19-24. DOI: 10.1097/00075197-200201000-00004

[52] Naughton C, Galvin R, McCullagh R, Horgan F. Comprehensive geriatric assessment-where are we now, where do we need to be in the context of global ageing? Age and Ageing. 2023;**52**(11):afad210. DOI: 10.1093/ageing/afad210

[53] Arakelyan S, Lone N, Anand A, et al. Effectiveness of holistic assessment-based interventions in improving outcomes in adults with multiple long-term conditions and/or frailty: An umbrella review protocol. JBI Evidence Synthesis. 2023;**21**(9):1863-1878. DOI: 10.11124/JBIES-22-00406

[54] Veniero D, Strüber D, Thut G, Herrmann CS. Noninvasive brain stimulation techniques can modulate cognitive processing. Organizational Research Methods. 2019;**22**(1):116-147. DOI: 10.1177/1094428116658960

[55] Woods AJ, Antal A, Bikson M, Boggio PS, Brunoni AR, Celnik P, et al. A technical guide to tDCS, and related non-invasive brain stimulation tools. Clinical Neurophysiology. 2016;**127**:1031-1048

[56] Klink K, Paßmann S, Kasten FH, Peter J. The modulation of cognitive performance with transcranial alternating current stimulation: A systematic review of frequency-specific effects. Brain Sciences. 2020;**10**(12):932. DOI: 10.3390/brainsci10120932

[57] Lefaucheur JP, André-Obadia N, Antal A, Ayache SS, Baeken C, Benninger DH, et al. Evidence-based guidelines on the therapeutic use of repetitive transcranial magnetic stimulation (rTMS). Clinical Neurophysiology. 2014;**125**(11):2150-2206

[58] Mateos-Aparicio P, Rodríguez-Moreno A. The impact of studying brain plasticity. Frontiers in Cellular Neuroscience. 2019;**13**:66. DOI: 10.3389/fncel.2019.00066

[59] Cope EC, Gould E. Adult neurogenesis, glia, and the extracellular matrix. Cell Stem Cell. 2019;**24**(5):690-705. DOI: 10.1016/j.stem.2019.03.023

[60] Cameron HA, Glover LR. Adult neurogenesis: Beyond learning and memory. Annual Review of Psychology. 2015;**66**:53-81. DOI: 10.1146/annurev-psych-010814-015006

[61] Andersen N, Krauth N, Nabavi S. Hebbian plasticity in vivo: Relevance and induction. Current Opinion in Neurobiology. 2017;**45**:188-192. DOI: 10.1016/j.conb.2017.06.001

[62] Culig L, Chu X, Bohr VA. Neurogenesis in aging and age-related neurodegenerative diseases. Ageing Research Reviews. 2022;**78**:101636. DOI: 10.1016/j.arr.2022.101636

[63] Tatti E, Rossi S, Innocenti I, Rossi A, Santarnecchi E. Non-invasive brain stimulation of the aging brain: State of the art and future perspectives. Ageing Research Reviews. 2016;**29**:66-89. DOI: 10.1016/j.arr.2016.05.006

[64] Goldthorpe RA, Rapley JM, Violante IR. A systematic review of non-invasive brain stimulation applications to memory in healthy aging. Frontiers in Neurology. 2020;**11**:575075. DOI: 10.3389/fneur.2020.575075

Chapter 3

Utilization of Comprehensive Geriatric Assessment (P3G) in Primary Health Center at Medan City and Deli Serdang District of North Sumatera Province Indonesia

Elman Boy, Alfi Syahri Pinem, Aulia Ulfa, Bonita Iravany Putri, Devi Pahlawati, Ivando Adedra, Krisna Syahputra Hutapea, Raudatul Popy Ramadani, Retno Pertiwi, Rika Karim Chan and Ulil Amri Saragih

Abstract

The Ministry of Health of the Republic of Indonesia has issued Comprehensive Geriatric Assessment (P3G) guidelines in 2017, but data regarding its use in health care institutions are still limited. Community health centers as the spearhead of primary care always accept geriatric patients and should utilize CGA. The objective is to find out the results of using a comprehensive assessment guide for geriatric patients at the Medan City Health Center and Deli Serdang Regency Health Center in 2018. This research was conducted using a descriptive method with a cross-sectional design, the respondents taken were elderly people seeking treatment at three health centers, namely Sukaramai Health Center, Medan City, Bandar Khalipah Health Center and Tanjung Rejo Health Center, Deli Serdang Regency in the period August and September 2018. The number of respondents was taken using the Slovin method, data collection was carried out through questionnaire interviews and data analysis using SPSS. There were 120 respondents, 60.8% of respondents experienced mild- moderate dependence. In the IADL examination, 89.2% were still able to carry out activities independently. The results of checking the risk of falling showed that 57.5% of respondents experienced a low risk. On the GDS examination, 67.5% of respondents did not experience depression. In the Mini-Cog examination, 78% of respondents had normal cognitive function. On the MMSE examination, 80.8% of respondents' cognitive function was still normal. On the AMT examination, 73.3% of respondents did not experience memory problems. In the MNA screening examination, 66.7% of respondents did not have nutritional problems. Conclusion: Most of the elderly who come to the health center are in the age range 60–74 and still have good functional abilities.

Keywords: geriatrics, elderly, P3G, Community Health Center, Ministry of Health

1. Introduction

Elderly health maintenance aimed to keep the elderly healthy and productive socially and economically. For this reason, it is necessary to have health service facilities to facilitate the elderly so that they can live independently and productively socially and economically. Apart from the right to health, seniors also have the same rights in social, national and state life. Efforts to improve the welfare of the elderly are directed so that the elderly are still empowered so that they can play a role in development activities by taking into account the functions, skills, age and physical condition of the elderly [1].

One of the successful impacts of health development is the reduction in birth rates, morbidity and mortality rates as well as an increase in the life expectancy of the population. Based on data, Life Expectancy (UHH) in Indonesia has increased from time to time. From 68.6 years in 2004 to 70.6 years in 2010. In 2022 it will increase to 72 years. This condition resulted in an increase in the number of elderly people. According to the results of the 2010 Population Census, the elderly population in Indonesia is 18.04 million people or 7.6% of the total population. In 2025 it is estimated that the number of elderly people will increase to 36 million people [2].

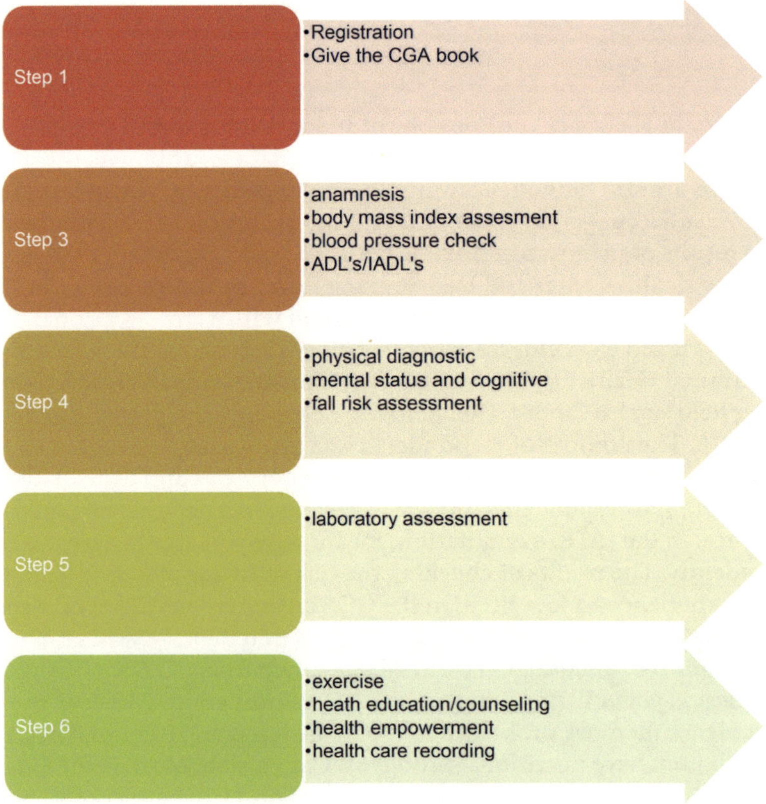

Figure 1.
Flow of services for elderly patients in primary care health facilities.

The increasing number of elderly people will also affect the number of dependency burdens. The old dependency ratio is a number that indicates the degree of dependence of the elderly on the productive age population. This figure is a comparison between the number of elderly people (60 years and over) and the number of productive people (15–59 years). To reduce the burden of dependency, the efforts made so that the elderly can live independently and remain productive must be increased. Naturally the process of getting old causes a person to experience physical and mental, spiritual, economic and social changes. One of the very basic problems in the elderly is health problems so that health coaching is needed in the pre-elderly and elderly groups, even from an early age (**Figure 1**) [3].

Primary health care facilities as the leading unit in public and individual health services are available in all districts and even every village in Indonesia. In this regard, Primary Health Service Facilities are expected to be able to carry out promotive, preventive, curative and rehabilitative efforts and hospital transition care for the elderly [4]. Elderly health services in Primary Health Care Facilities must be carried out in a professional and quality manner, complete, integrated and integrated with due regard to the elderly aspects of the elderly [5].

The Ministry of Health of the Republic of Indonesia has published the 2017 Comprehensive Elderly Assessment (P3G) guidelines for use in comprehensive elderly health checks at first-level health care facilities. P3G is part of the Comprehensive Elderly Management (CGM) with a multidimensional assessment approach, in the form of medical, psychosocial, functional abilities and limitations of elderly patients. In general, Indonesian sociodemographics, the ratio of the percentage of elderly women is higher than that of men (53.3, 46.7). In order to improve the quality of elderly health services in primary health care facilities, a handbook for elderly health services is needed [6].

2. Elderly health services at primary health service facilities

Primary health service facilities are health service facilities that carry out community health efforts and individual health efforts at the first level, by prioritizing promotive and preventive efforts, to achieve the highest degree of public health in their working area [7]. The implementation of elderly health services in Primary Health Service Facilities is carried out in a comprehensive manner with the following principles [8]:

1. Providing good and quality service

2. Prioritize services for the elderly and provide safe and easily accessible facilities

3. Provide support/guidance to the elderly and their families on an ongoing basis in maintaining and improving their health, so that they remain healthy, independent and active

4. Carry out services proactively to be able to reach as many elderly targets as possible in the working area of the Primary Health Service Facilities through service activities outside the building;

5. Coordinating with cross-programs using a life cycle approach as one of the approaches to realizing healthy, independent and active elderly; And

6. Collaborating with cross-sectors, including social organizations and the business world on a partnership basis, to provide services and coaching in order to improve the quality of life for seniors.

7. Elderly services at Primary Health Care Facilities are provided to elderly patients in accordance with the competence of general practitioners at Primary Health Care Facilities

2.1 Definition of elderly

Elderly or geriatrics comes from the words geros (old) and iatrea (maintenance); so it is clear that the science of old age is part of medicine and gerontology which specifically studies health and diseases in the elderly. Elderly patient also refers to the condition that he is 60 years and over. Elderly patients have a number of characteristics that differentiate them from adults in general [9].

2.2 Elderly characteristics

Elderly patients have several characteristics, namely multipathology, atypical appearance of symptoms and signs, decreased physiological reserve, usually accompanied by impaired functional status and in Indonesia generally with nutritional disorders. Multipathology refers to the notion that an elderly patient has more than one disease at the same time. The diseases he suffers are usually accumulations of degenerative diseases that have been attached to him for years and due to certain acute conditions result in the patient having to be hospitalized or being forced to lie at home (bedridden). This multipathological condition causes the symptoms and signs that appear in a patient to be unclear [10].

2.3 Symptoms and signs

signs and symptoms of elderly patients are usually not typical. For example, an elderly patient with pneumonia rarely shows the full range of symptoms, such as fever, cough, shortness of breath and leukocytosis. Symptoms that often appear are loss of appetite, general weakness and on physical examination, disturbances of consciousness such as apathy or delirium can be seen. Likewise, elderly patients with a premorbid history of osteoarthritis in several large joints who have congestive heart failure, often come to the emergency department with complaints of 'falling'. On further anamnesis, there were no complaints of shortness of breath, dyspnoea d'effort or paroxysmal nocturnal dyspnea. In addition to changes in consciousness and 'falls', the presenting symptoms of elderly patients are often milder than the actual severe condition.

Due to the course of age, the function of the elderly organs will decrease. This decrease in physiology will have the consequence of decreasing the reserve power of the physiology. For example, an elderly patient suffering from pneumonia is usually accompanied by decreased non-specific immune systems such as decreased respiratory ciliary activity and cough reflex. Both of these make it impossible for elderly patients to be treated only with antibiotics and mucolytics; several efforts are needed to increase the non-specific resistance of the body such as tapping, breathing exercises and postural drainage. Another example, for example, is a decrease in the number of kidney glomeruli that causes drug administration in elderly patients to require consideration of dose adjustments (because drug excretion is mostly through the kidneys) [11].

Elderly patients also often come for treatment with impaired nutritional status. Malnutrition is often not noticed by patients and their families until the patient actually falls into a state of poor nutrition. Body mass index describes nutritional status more accurately. Deficiency of vitamins and minerals often accompanies undernutrition and malnutrition [12].

These various characteristics cause a doctor or nurse to have high sensitivity in compiling a list of diagnoses or a list of patient health problems in order of priority. A medical diagnosis alone will not adequately describe the patient's health problems. Conditions of immobilization, inability to transfer the body independently, difficulty eating, communication disorders are some examples of health problems that often escape medical diagnosis, even though they greatly affect the overall success of treatment [13].

2.4 Principles of management of elderly patients

In the management of health problems in the elderly, it is necessary to pay attention to the characteristics of elderly patients that can affect clinical appearance, the management program provided, including drug administration, as well as the risks of potential complications. Functional status is a very useful monitoring tool in assessing the severity of the disease and the success of treatment [14].

2.5 Principles of drug administration

Starting from a low dose and increasing gradually until you get the desired effect (Start Low and Go Slow), except for giving antibiotics. As far as possible the patient should not take too much medicine; even though there is no agreement on the term polypharmacy itself, at least if there is one type of drug that is not properly indicated then monitoring of adverse effects should be carried out. The more drugs consumed, the higher the iatrogenic risk that may occur. It often happens that patients submit subjective complaints which turn out to be side effects of the drugs given, so doctors must carry out periodic reviews of the drugs the patient is taking [14].

2.6 Pharmacokinetics

Drug pharmacokinetics greatly influence the effect of treatment in elderly patients. A decrease in the composition of body fluids and an increase in the central fat component will affect the concentration of the drug in the target organs. For drugs that are fat soluble (lipophilic), they will be dissolved and bound longer in tissues (especially the central nervous system) thereby extending the half-life; the clinical implication is that the dose of lipophilic drugs should be sparing. For water-soluble (hydrophilic) drugs, the concentration in plasma will increase so that the dose needs to be lowered [15].

Drug metabolism occurs in the liver via conjugation or oxidation pathways [16]. Oxidation pathways that use cytochrome P-450 enzymes will experience a decrease in activity with increasing age. So that drugs that will be metabolized through this pathway need to pay attention to the amount of dose. The conjugation pathway usually does not decrease in activity as a person ages. Once metabolized, the drug will be excreted through the kidneys. The number of glomeruli and kidney function will gradually decrease according to a person's age so that drugs that are excreted only through the kidneys have a risk of accumulation. Drugs that besides having renal and liver (bile) excretion pathways will have a lower risk [14].

2.7 Pharmacodynamics

After the drug enters the blood circulation it will be bound to albumin. Each drug has a different affinity for albumin. The higher the affinity, the lower the concentration in plasma and the lower the binding to albumin, the higher the free level in plasma. This will affect the distribution and pharmacodynamics or drug effects in body tissues [14].

3. Health services for the elderly

Health services for the elderly who come to the Primary Health Care Facilities should be provided in a special room so that the elderly do not have to queue together with other public patients. However, if the condition of the Primary Health Service Facility is not possible, it can be carried out in the general examination room with the condition that elderly patients must be prioritized [5].

4. Comprehensive geriatric assessment

Every elderly who visits a primary health care facility on their first visit or contact with a health worker will carry out a plenary assessment program using the Comprehensive Geriatric Assessment or Pengkajian Paripurna Pasien Geritri (P3G), which is an interdisciplinary diagnostic process, to determine medical problems and capabilities, functional abilities, psychosocial and environment for elderly patients. Because the characteristics and syndromes in elderly patients are different, a special bio-psycho-social oriented approach is needed for each elderly patient which is absolutely necessary for complete management [6].

This plenary assessment itself is a basic instrument that must be owned by every doctor, nurse, nutritionist, physical therapist and others who manage elderly patients according to their respective competencies. With P3G health workers carry out a thorough assessment of the elderly from biological, cognitive, psychological and social aspects to determine management problems for the elderly and plan according to the needs and available manpower can be added. P3G is carried out by a team led by a doctor with other members namely nurses, nutrition workers, and trained community health workers [17].

Completeness in question is actually not only limited to what must be studied but also concerns other aspects. These aspects are: doctors do not only carry out treatment (curative aspect) but also need to carry out various disease prevention, as well as prevention of complications (preventing decubitus, preventing deep vein thrombosis in immobilization cases). The next aspect is taking a rehabilitative approach for cases with disabilities, for example coughing disorders, expectoration disorders of sputum, swallowing disorders and position change disorders. In the end, doctors must also make promotive efforts such as maintaining range of motion in immobilization, stimulating physical and mental activity, increasing family knowledge about caring for elderly patients at home and so on [18].

4.1 Elements of elderly plenary assessment in primary health care facilities

Elderly patients must be managed according to lege artis rules. In the identity component, in addition to personal identity, economic, social, environmental issues must also be asked, with whom the patient lives or who is the closest person to contact if something happens, etc. In the anamnesis component, in addition to the main complaints and medical history, a history of surgery, medical history (both from doctors and over-the-counter drugs), family history of illness, simple nutritional history and system history should be asked. System anamnesis is very important because often the main complaint is not in accordance with the main problem which is the priority of management (which is life threatening). In addition, it is very likely that the elderly and elderly patients will not express their complaints unless asked [19].

4.2 Vital signs examination

Examination of vital signs is highly recommended to really pay attention to the degree of decrease or change in consciousness (if any). Examination of blood pressure and heart rate should be done in a lying position and sitting and standing (if possible); Orthostatic hypotension is more common in elderly patients [20].

4.3 Physical examination

The physical examination is carried out according to the systematics of the organ systems starting from the cardiovascular system, respiratory system, gastrointestinal system, genitourinary system, musculoskeletal system, hematological system, endocrinology metabolic system and neurologic examination [21].

4.4 Nutritional status assessment

Assessment of nutritional status begins with early detection using MNA, followed by recording nutritional intake, measuring BMI (if the patient can still stand upright), or measuring fathom length, knee height, or sitting height (if the patient cannot stand straight). Mini Nutritional Assessment (MNA) is one of the instruments to detect the risk of malnutrition or the presence of malnutrition in the elderly group. Examination with the MNA Instrument consists of two stages, namely the first stage (screening), and the second stage (assessment). If the score in the first stage <11, will proceed to the second stage. Furthermore, a person is classified as: malnourished if the total score is <17, and at risk of malnutrition if the total score is between 17–23.5 [22].

Body mass index (BMI) or Quetelet index is a method used to determine a person's nutritional status. BMI is a prediction bodyhuman based on a person's weight and height. The ideal normal standard used for people mature aged over 20 years is BMI between 18.5 to 24.9. A person is said to be overweight if the BMI is between 25.0 and 29.9. If BMI < 18.5 means underweight and BMI ≥30 means obesity [23].

In some cases, BMI can help doctors determine a person's overall health status and risk of developing chronic disease. But, still doctorit is not only possible to rely on BMI as a consideration factor because BMI is not completely a reliable assessment for every different body type. BMI figures need to be known because they can be a signal about a person's health condition. A low BMI can indicate that someone has it malnutrition. It is possible that his body is not capable of absorption nutrition well or the person is not getting intake calories sufficient to support its activities. Conversely, if the BMI number is higher, it indicates that a person is at risk heart disease, diabetes and cancer higher than someone with a normal BMI. Knowing this, doctors can refer patient on dietitian registered to help patients achieve their ideal body weight and reduce the risk of developing various health problems [24].

4.5 Functional status check

Examination of functional status is intended to determine a person's ability to carry out activities of daily living independently. For example, getting up from a lying position, sitting, walking, bathing, urinating, dressing, preening, eating, going up and down stairs and defecating. Due to the acute illness that attacks, usually elderly patients will experience a decrease in functional status, for example from independent to mild or moderate dependence, from mild dependence to moderate to severe dependence, even total dependence. In determining the degree of dependence of a person, it should be noted that the data obtained from direct information must be adjusted to data from the family living with the patient as well as from direct observation by health workers. Determination of this functional status must be done carefully, preferably by involving the family and being observed alone. The determination needs to be made several times to evaluate the progress or setbacks that may occur [25].

Functional status was examined using Barthel's ADL index and Lawton's Instrumental Activities of Daily Living (IADL). The Barthel scale is ordinal scale used to measure ability to perform daily life activities or activities of daily living (ADL). Each activity item is scored on this scale with a number of points assigned to each level or rating. ADL uses ten variables that describe a person's mobility. A higher number is associated with a greater likelihood of being able to live at home more independently. *Instrumental Activities of Daily Living (IADL) Lawton* useful for assessing a person's ability to perform daily tasks such as using the telephone, washing clothes, and handling finances. The IADL measures eight domains, can be assigned within 10–15 min [26].

4.6 Fall risk assessment in elderly patients

Fall is defined as a sudden, uncontrolled, unintentional displacement of the body onto the ground or other object. A near fall is a sudden loss of balance that does not result in a fall or other injury. This can include a person who slips or trips but is able to regain control before the fall. Based on existing data, the incidence of falls in the elderly is increasing from year to year, which is caused by environmental factors and illnesses. Therefore, it is necessary to carry out prevention efforts by assessing the risk of falling in elderly patients using the above instruments. To carry out a fall risk assessment, it can be done by using the Fall Risk Assessment questionnaire for Elderly Patients. Medical personnel need to identify the symptoms/criteria as stated in the questionnaire. If the patient has these symptoms/criteria, then the patient gets a score according to the scale listed.

If not, then the patient gets a value of 0.

Furthermore, all scores are summed up and classified according to the level of risk, namely:

- Low risk if score 1–3 Perform low risk interventions

- High risk if score $\geq$ 4 Perform high risk interventions

Patients with a high risk of falling should be given a fall prevention program in the form of:

1. Give the patient a bracelet indicating the risk of falling that is worn when the patient is in a public facility

2. Egrief prevents falls in patients and families.

3. Patients at high risk of falling should be referred to a physician trained in geriatrics for further management.

4. Treatments that can be given are: addressing the risk factors found include:

    a. Using overcome: where this is caused by hypertension so hypertension needs to be controlled more regularly

    b. Visual disturbances (cataracts) are treated by being referred to an ophthalmologist for cataract surgery

    c. Strengthen muscle strength with training

4.7 Supporting examinations, carried out as needed

From the results of the plenary assessment, the elderly will then be divided into several groups:

1. Seniors are healthy and independent;

2. Healthy seniors with mild dependence;

3. Healthy elderly with moderate dependency;

4. Elderly with heavy/total dependency;

5. Post-hospital elderly (first two weeks);

6. Seniors who need nutritional care; or

7. Seniors in need accompaniment (having psycho-cognitive problems).

Based on these groups, appropriate programs for the elderly will be carried out, including:

Group a (healthy and independent elderly) and group b (healthy elderly with mild dependence) can directly participate in the Elderly program in a certain room.

Elderly belonging to group c (healthy elderly with moderate dependence) and group d (elderly with severe/total dependence) must take part in a home care service program if necessary involving caregivers or possibly need to be referred to hospital.

For group e (elderly after first two weeks of treatment), group f (elderly who need nutritional care), and group g (elderly who need assistance, have psycho-cognitive problems) with independent functional status can be served in the activity room, while the elderly with a mild to moderate degree of dependence must be monitored by a doctor while participating in the program in the activity room [27].

4.8 Assessment of psychosocial status

Assessment of the psychosocial status of the elderly experiencing various psychological problems that need to be considered by doctors, nurses, families and health workers. Handling problems early will help the elderly in implementing problem-solving strategies. Changes in psychosocial status that often occur in the elderly are mature, dependent, self hater, angry, arrogant, and others [28].

4.9 Social status assessment

Assessment of social status is to assess the treatment of people around the elderly who are very influential on the physical and mental health conditions of the elderly such as mistreatment/abuse, and neglect of the elderly (neglected). In addition, an assessment of social status can find family potential that can be utilized to help the patient's recovery [29].

4.10 Services for healthy seniors

Cognitive status examination is a screening for dementia (senility); the simplest modality is Abbreviated Mental Test (AMT), categorizing it into mild, moderate and severe cognitive impairment. To check cognitive status can also be assessed by Mini Cog and clock drawing test. Dementia is a condition of continuous progressive mental function decline, getting worse over time, including decreased memory of things that have just happened, decline in language proficiency, intellectual decline (thinking power), which interferes with daily activities and is generally accompanied by changes in behavior and personality. The two most common types of dementia are dementia of the Alzheimer's type and vascular (post-stroke) dementia.

decreased short-term memory (recent memory), thinking power, value power, orientation abilities, language skills and other cognitive functions. the patient often appears apathetic or indifferent, but may appear alert and reasonable, despite poor memory. Decreased function of basic daily activities (dressing, bathing, cooking, etc.) Loss of emotional control: easily confused, prone to crying or easily offended (angry). Examination of memory and thinking power, can be done in several ways, including:

Mini Cog: the ability to recall the names of three objects immediately after saying them and after a while (approx. 3 min). examination of the clock drawing test or clock drawing test (CDT). AMT test examination. MMSE examination. Note: If the situation is not possible then one of the instruments above can be selected [30].

5. Research finding

5.1 Research on the description of a complete study of geriatric patients at the Medan City Health Center and Deli Serdang Regency in 2018

A descriptive study with a cross-sectional design, determining the number of respondents using the Slovin formula and using the Comprehensive Geriatric

Category	Subcategory	Count	Percentage
Sample size		120	100
Sex	Male	56	46.7
	Female	64	53.3
Age	Elderly (60–74 years old)	109	90.8
	Old (75–90 years old)	10	8.3
	Very old (>90 years old)	1	0.9

Table 1.
Characteristics of respondents.

Assessment questionnaire instrument. The authors conducted this by involving several primary health care facilities in two districts and cities, namely Medan City and Deli Serdang District, North Sumatra Province. The research population is the elderly aged ≥ 60 years. who went to Primary Health Facilities in 2018 involving 120 elderly respondents. the study was carried out for six months. The study population was elderly aged ≥ 60 years. who went to the Sukaramai District Health Office in Medan City, Bandar Khalipah Primary health center Deli Serdang district and Tanjung Rejo Primary health center Deli Serdang district on 27 August 2018–20 September 2018.

Sociodemographics, it was found that the ratio of elderly women was higher than that of men (53.3% :46.7%). Statistics in Indonesia state that the elderly population over 60 years is dominated by women compared to men. The sociodemographics of the respondents were 60–74 years (90%), 75–90 years (8.3%) and >90 years old (0.9%) (**Table 1**).

ADL examination showed the results of respondents with a mild-moderate dependence level of 61%, 37% were independent and 2% were totally dependent. Based on the IADL examination, it was found that the independent level was 89.2%. Based on the examination of the risk of falling in this study, it was found that 54.2% had a low risk of falling. Research confirms that in patients who come for treatment at Primary Health Care Facilities are still able to walk on their own. However, this study did not confirm whether the respondent came alone or was accompanied by his family for treatment at a primary health facility.

Based on the GDS examination, in this study 62.5% did not experience depressive disorders. One of the factors that supports the high number of elderly people without depression in this study can be caused by high social activity and interpersonal relationships among fellow residents. Where residents work together and interact in everyday life. Getting high social and environmental support will make the elderly feel more comfortable and happier, so that they can keep them from the risk of depression.

Based on the Mini-Cog examination in this study, 73.3% did not experience a decrease in cognitive impairment. Based on the MMSE examination, in this study it was found that 83.5% of respondents did not experience cognitive impairment. Based on the AMT examination in this study, it was found that 77.1% did not experience memory impairment/normal. Based on the MNA examination, in this study it was found that 66.7% were in the category of good nutrition and the risk category of undernutrition was 33.3% [6] (**Table 2**).

Category	**Age**			
	60–74 (%)	**75–90 (%)**	**>90 (%)**	**Total (%)**
ADL				
Independent	38.5	30	0	37.5
Mild Moderate Dependence	61.5	60	0	60.8
Total Care	0	10	100	1.7
IADL				
Unable to do at all	0	0	0.8	0.8
Need help all the time	0	0.8	0	0.8
Need some help	7.5	1.7	0	9.2
Independent	83	5.8	0	89
Total care				
Risk of falling				
No risk	9	0	0	9
Low risk	65	4	0	69
High risk	35	6	1	42
GDS				
Normal	75	6	0	81
Probable depression	34	4	1	39
Indicative of depression	0	0	0	0
Mini Cog				
Normal	88	6	0	94
Probable cognitive impairment	21	4	1	26
MMSE				
Normal	91	6	0	97
Mild cognitive impairment	17	3	0	20
Severe cognitive impairment	1	1	1	3
AMT				
Normal	84	4	0	88
Moderate impairment	25	6	1	32
MNA				
Normal	76	4	0	80
At risk	33	6	1	40

Table 2.
Frequency distribution of comprehensive geriatric assessment.

DOI: http://dx.doi.org/10.5772/intechopen.112596

Author details

Elman Boy*, Alfi Syahri Pinem, Aulia Ulfa, Bonita Iravany Putri, Devi Pahlawati, Ivando Adedra, Krisna Syahputra Hutapea, Raudatul Popy Ramadani, Retno Pertiwi, Rika Karim Chan and Ulil Amri Saragih
Department of Public Health of Medical Faculty of Universitas Muhammadiyah Sumatera Utara, Indonesia

*Address all correspondence to: elmanboy@umsu.ac.id

References

[1] Kuroiwa S, Kita K, Kuroiwa M, Minami S, Yamashiro S. Home and social role as factors that lead to the maintenance of health in the elderly: A Longitudinal Study. SSRN Electronic Journal. 2022. DOI: 10.2139/ssrn.4235880

[2] Kristanto E, Daerobi A, Samudro BR. Indonesian life expectancy: Role of health infrastructure and socio-economic status. Signifikan Journal of Ilmu Ekon. 2019;**8**:159-178. DOI: 10.15408/sjie.v8i1.9579

[3] Lee W-J, Peng L-N, Lin C-H, Chen R-C, Lin S-Z, Loh C-H, et al. Effects of incorporating multidomain interventions into integrated primary care on quality of life: A randomised controlled trial. Lancet Health Longevity. 2021;**2**:e712-e723. DOI: 10.1016/S2666-7568(21)00248-8

[4] de Menezes TM, de Oliveira AL, Santos LB, de Freitas RA, Pedreira LC, SMCB V. Hospital transition care for the elderly: an integrative review. Revista Brasileira de Enfermagem. 2019;**72**:294-301. DOI: 10.1590/0034-7167-2018-0286

[5] Lubenow JAM, Silva AO. What the elderly think of the care provided by health services. Rev Bras Geriatr e Gerontol. 2019:22. DOI: 10.1590/1981-22562019022.180195

[6] Boy E, Pinem AS, Ulfa A, Putri BI, Pahlawati D, Adedra I, et al. Utilization of comprehensive geriatric assessment (P3G) in primary health center at Medan City and Deli Serdang District of North Sumatera Province Indonesia 2018. International Journal of Human Health Science. 2019;**3**:88. DOI: 10.31344/ijhhs.v3i2.82

[7] He AJ, Tang VFY. Integration of health services for the elderly in Asia: A scoping review of Hong Kong, Singapore, Malaysia, Indonesia. Health Policy (New York). 2021;**125**:351-362. DOI: 10.1016/j.healthpol.2020.12.020

[8] Garrard JW, Cox NJ, Dodds RM, Roberts HC, Sayer AA. Comprehensive geriatric assessment in primary care: a systematic review. Aging Clinical and Experimental Research. 2020;**32**:197-205. DOI: 10.1007/s40520-019-01183-w

[9] Türkbeyler İH, Öztürk ZA, Göl M, Abiyev A, Kaya B, Atakur S, et al. What is geriatrics? Geriatrics or older adults health and diseases? European Journal of Geriatric Gerontology. 2019;**1**:51-55. DOI: 10.4274/ejgg.galenos.2019.92

[10] Gw E. The neurological, multisystemic, polygenomic and multipathological basis of aging (the 'Autonomic' Hypothesis). Journal of Neurology and Neurobiology. 2020;**6**. DOI: 10.16966/2379-7150.164

[11] Evers BM, Townsend CM, Thompson JC. Organ physiology of aging. The Surgical Clinics of North America. 1994;**74**:23-39. DOI: 10.1016/S0039-6109(16)46226-2

[12] Besora-Moreno M, Llauradó E, Tarro L, Solà R. Social and economic factors and malnutrition or the risk of malnutrition in the elderly: A systematic review and meta-analysis of observational studies. Nutrients. 2020;**12**:737. DOI: 10.3390/nu12030737

[13] Shi Y, Fan F, Zhang Z. Simulation of performance evaluation model for medical-elderly care integrated institutions based on system dynamics. BMC Health Services Research. 2022;**22**:1451. DOI: 10.1186/s12913-022-08835-0

[14] Stuhec M, Bratović N,Mrhar A. Impact of clinical pharmacist's interventions on pharmacotherapy management in elderly patients on polypharmacy with mental health problems including quality of life: A prospective non-randomized study. Scientific Reports. 2019;**9**:16856. DOI: 10.1038/s41598-019-53057-w

[15] Drenth-van Maanen AC, Wilting I, Jansen PAF. Prescribing medicines to older people—How to consider the impact of ageing on human organ and body functions. British Journal of Clinical Pharmacology. 2020;**86**:1921-1930. DOI: 10.1111/bcp.14094

[16] Li Y, Meng Q, Yang M, Liu D, Hou X, Tang L, et al. Current trends in drug metabolism and pharmacokinetics. Acta Pharmaceutica Sinica B. 2019;**9**:1113-1144. DOI: 10.1016/j.apsb.2019.10.001

[17] Keli A, Gondodiputro S, Arisanti N. Implementation of comprehensive geriatric assessment in elderly-friendly Public Health Centers and General Public Health Centers in Bandung. Althea Medical Journal. 2020;**7**:65-71. DOI: 10.15850/amj.v7n2.1923

[18] Rudnicka E, Napierała P, Podfigurna A, Męczekalski B, Smolarczyk R, Grymowicz M. The World Health Organization (WHO) approach to healthy ageing. Maturitas. 2020;**139**:6-11. DOI: 10.1016/j.maturitas.2020.05.018

[19] Kim E, Kim S, Rhee J. A study on model of psychotherapy narration focused on mental well-being for stress management in the elderly. Sustainability. 2023;**15**:2656. DOI: 10.3390/su15032656

[20] Ahmed N, Greenberg P. Examining outcomes in cases of elderly patients who fell from ground level at home with normal vital signs at the scene: An analysis of the National Trauma Data Bank. Journal of Trauma and Acute Care Surgery. 2019;**87**:672-677. DOI: 10.1097/TA.0000000000002400

[21] Monteiro MCD, da Martins MM, Schoeller SD. Evaluation of the health level of the elderly: Patient care team considerations. Revista Brasileira de Enfermagem. 2022:75. DOI: 10.1590/0034-7167-2020-1277

[22] Loddo S, Salis F, Rundeddu S, Serchisu L, Peralta MM, Mandas A. Nutritional status and potentially inappropriate medications in elderly. Journal of Clinical Medicine. 2022;**11**:3465. DOI: 10.3390/jcm11123465

[23] Trevisan C, Crippa A, Ek S, Welmer A-K, Sergi G, Maggi S, et al. Nutritional status, body mass index, and the risk of falls in community-dwelling older adults: A systematic review and meta-analysis. Journal of the American Medical Directors Association. 2019;**20**:569-582.e7. DOI: 10.1016/j.jamda.2018.10.027

[24] Abd Aziz NAS, Mohd Fahmi Teng NI, Kamarul ZM. Geriatric nutrition risk index is comparable to the mini nutritional assessment for assessing nutritional status in elderly hospitalized patients. Clinical Nutrition ESPEN. 2019;**29**:77-85. DOI: 10.1016/j.clnesp.2018.12.002

[25] Oliveira A, Nossa P, Mota-Pinto A. Assessing functional capacity and factors determining functional decline in the elderly: A cross-sectional study. Acta Médica Portuguesa. 2019;**32**:654-660. DOI: 10.20344/amp.11974

[26] Beltz S, Gloystein S, Litschko T, Laag S, van den Berg N. Multivariate analysis of independent determinants of ADL/IADL and quality of life in the elderly. BMC Geriatrics. 2022;**22**:894. DOI: 10.1186/s12877-022-03621-3

[27] Kim J, Lee W, Lee SH. A systematic review of the guidelines and Delphi study for the multifactorial fall risk assessment of community-dwelling elderly. International Journal of Environmental Research and Public Health. 2020;**17**:6097. DOI: 10.3390/ijerph17176097

[28] Lee K, Jeong G-C, Yim J. Consideration of the psychological and mental health of the elderly during COVID-19: A theoretical review. International Journal of Environmental Research and Public Health. 2020;**17**:8098. DOI: 10.3390/ijerph17218098

[29] Agarwalla R, Saikia A, Baruah R. Assessment of the nutritional status of the elderly and its correlates. Journal of Family and Community Medicine. 2015;**22**:39. DOI: 10.4103/2230-8229.149588

[30] Banjongrewadee M, Wongpakaran N, Wongpakaran T, Pipanmekaporn T, Punjasawadwong Y, Mueankwan S. The role of perceived stress and cognitive function on the relationship between neuroticism and depression among the elderly: A structural equation model approach. BMC Psychiatry. 2020;**20**:25. DOI: 10.1186/s12888-020-2440-9

Chapter 4

Frailty, Polypill and Quality of Life in Elderly

Sunil Kumar and Nishtha Manuja

Abstract

Frailty is an age-related state of increased susceptibility of functional decline that may be reversed or at least slowed progressiveness. It is characterized by impairments in a number of physiological systems and is linked to a higher risk of morbidity or unexpected hospitalization. It is a newly recognized geriatric syndrome in clinical practice, and excess healthcare expenses from consultations, polypill use, and hospitalization are some of its correlations. When under stress, frailty results in a loss of autonomy in everyday activities and death. Elderly adults frequently have many comorbid ailments, which exposes them to multiple medications or polypill therapy. This is linked to a higher chance of negative drug reactions, which leads to more hospitalizations, high morbidity, mortality, and higher healthcare system costs. It's crucial to recognize these conditions in order to offer primary care patients early intervention and/or interdisciplinary management, which fits well with the physical and psychosocial model for their well-being.

Keywords: frailty, polypill, hospitalization, quality of life, prescription cascade

1. Introduction

The cutoff age for elderly is 60 years in the majority of nations, including India. Our society today considers the "young old" to be between 60 and 74 years old, the "middle old" to be between 75 and 84 years old, and the "old old" to be over 85 years old [1].

According to WHO, currently 1 in 10 people are 60 years or older; by 2050, that number will increase to 1 in 5 and 1 in 3 by 2150 [2]. One in five Europeans and one in every twenty Africans are 60 years of age or older. There will be less time to adapt to the effects of population ageing in developing countries because aging occurs more quickly there than in industrialized ones. Current global life expectancy is 66 years; however, in the least developed areas, males can expect only 14 years and women 16 years of additional life, respectively, while in the more developed areas, life expectancy at 60 is 18 years and 22 years, respectively [3]. India is home to more than 100 million senior people, according to the most recent census. Even though the number could rise to 170 million by 2025 and life expectancy would grow from the present 66–72 years, little is known about the health of this population and its medical needs.

In the years 2009–2013, women had a life expectancy at birth of 69.3 years compared to men's 65.8 years [4].

Frailty is a reduced physiological reserve of several organs that makes elderly people more vulnerable to shocks and more likely to experience negative outcomes [5]. The term "frail" is used to describe frail old individuals who are highly susceptible to unfavourable outcomes, such as falls, deteriorating disabilities, hospitalization, and mortality. Frailty, however, is not the same as old age or illness. When under stress, frailty results in a loss of autonomy in everyday activities and death. Physical weakness is thought to be potentially recoverable at this time. Due to the fact that frailty indices are beneficial for risk classification, forecasting the need for institutional care, and planning for necessary services, it is important to objectively detect frailty in aged individuals [2, 3].

In clinical practice and research, several frailty definitions and evaluation techniques have been created, and this has been the subject of many reviews and comparative studies [4, 5]. Particularly, Fried et al.'s frailty phenotype has gained recognition on a global scale. The fundamental benefit of Fried's approach is that it just calls for the evaluation of five factors: physical activity, grip strength, tiredness, and weight loss [4]. Although this is reasonable in terms of primary care, there is a problem with the way the measure was put together as non-frail, pre-frail, and frail.

The cumulative deficit model, which is based on a variety of factors including symptoms, signs, diseases, disabilities, and abnormal test values, together known as deficits, determines frailty [6]. The initial model had 92 variables, but later research has shown that this may be cut down to around 30 more manageable variables without losing predictive validity [7]. The variables can be used to create a frailty index (FI) score, which is a straightforward computation of each variable's presence or absence as a percentage of the whole.

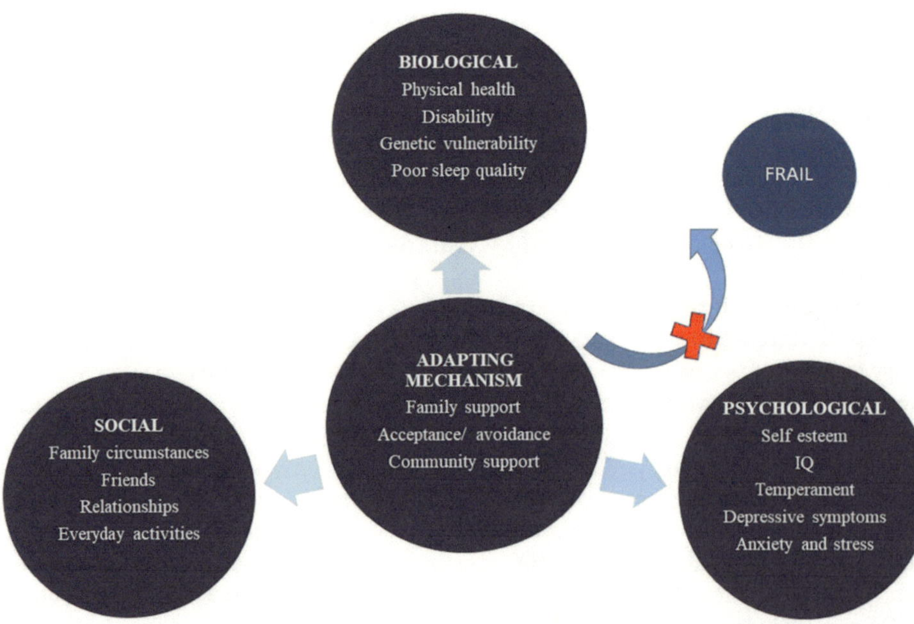

Figure 1.
Biopsychosocial factors associated with fraility.

In order to manage cases at the primary care level based on the concept of frailty, which fits well with the physical and psychosocial model, research should be conducted with the goal of identifying at-risk groups of elderly people in order to provide early intervention and/or multidisciplinary case management [8]. This ideal has, however, made it clear that there aren't any frailty measurements that are suitable for use in basic care. In fact, general practitioners still require simple tools for detecting frailty.

The biopsychosocial factors are also associated with complexities of the frailty that interrelate and lead to clinical and functional manifestations in older adults. These factors are interlaced with each other as shown in **Figure 1**. In biological component, physical health, disability, genetic vulnerability and poor sleep quality account for major factors. In social component- family circumstances, friends, relationships. And in psychological, self-esteem and anxiety are important factors.

2. Frailty: definition and pathophysiology

The term "frail" is used to describe frail old individuals who are highly susceptible to unfavorable outcomes, such as falls, deteriorating disabilities, hospitalization, and mortality. Frailty, however, is not the same as old age or illness. Therefore, even for patients with advanced single- or multi-organ disease processes, frailty, as a way to summarize health status, could provide additional relevant clinical information. Frailty is characterized by a need for assistance with daily living activities (ADLs), such as dressing, feeding, bathing, using the restroom, and moving around. Frailty and impairment usually coexist, and the likelihood is higher as age rises. The scenario could get more complex due to cognitive impairment [9].

Fried et al.'s definition of frailty syndrome, which includes three or more of the following symptoms: weakness, slow walking speed, self-reported weariness, limited physical activity, and unintended weight loss, is the most frequently accepted [2].

Abnormalities in numerous physiological and biochemical systems have been linked to fragility. These include low levels of insulin-like growth factor-1 and dehydroepiandrosterone-sulfate, anemia, low albumin, higher levels of inflammatory markers, particularly interleukin-6 and tumour necrosis factor, high hemoglobinA1c, and nutritional deficiencies. However, new research has shown that rather than a single biomarker, frailty is most closely linked to a mix of immunological and physiological abnormalities. This is in line with the theory that aging is the result of a complex system suffering a cumulative loss of redundancy over time. The likelihood of frailty appears to depend more on a critical mass of anomalies than on any single mechanism.

3. Elderly and disability

Although aging is largely a reflection of people living longer and generally in better health, it is also linked to chronic and degenerative diseases, which are more prevalent as people get older. Disability can negatively affect elderly people's quality of life and is a significant health marker that can have a huge social impact due to recurrent institutionalization and higher medical care. Additionally, as age increases, their chances of becoming disabled increases, and their chances of recovering from disability diminish [10]. The phrase "disability and elderly" covers a wide range of conditions, each with their own specific needs.

The International Classification of Functioning, Disability and Health (ICF) classifies impairments, activity limitations, and participation restrictions under the general heading of disability [11]. A constraint or lack of capacity to do a task in the manner or within the parameters deemed typical for a human being has been classified as a disability [12]. "Types of disability" are frequently characterized using just one component of disability, such as sensory, physical, mental, or intellectual impairments. Other times, health issues are confused with disability [12, 13].

Elderly people with disabilities can be divided into three categories: those who can manage their daily activities with the aids, those who have multiple health issues and severe limitations in their mental and/or physical functioning and need very high levels of care, and those who are functionally disabled in one or two activities of daily lifes or have mild cognitive impairments [14]. There is proof that older populations are more likely to experience several comorbidities, which can result in disability [15]. It has been well established in numerous studies from India that morbidity affects the physical functioning and psychological well-being of elderly populations; the necessity "to develop geriatric health care services in developing countries on the basis of existing morbidity profile" must be emphasized [16, 17]. Elderly people have been found to exhibit a variety of morbidity patterns, including hypertension, diabetes, arthritis, constipation, cataracts, and hearing loss, dyspepsia/heartburn, backache, dyspnoea, syncope, altered bowel habits, and blurring of vision. However, studies had lacked a clear definition of disability and were unable to quantify the impact of advancing age and associated morbid conditions as its main etiologies [16].

4. Frailty and falls

Any geriatric condition is more likely to manifest in weak older persons, and there is growing evidence that links frailty especially to falls. A framework for examining why and how the frail older person is at danger of falling is provided by viewing frailty as the breakdown bipedal ambulation, which requires neurological control of different muscles on joints with sensory feedback signals and commands from the motor cortex. Therefore, it should not come as a surprise when weak people (who are equivalent to a system that has lost redundancy) experience falls because they become unable to integrate various inputs in the face of seemingly insignificant stressors.

It is important to note that the fall is not a diagnosis but can be a manifestation of "multiple underlying disease like visual impairment (cataract, corneal opacity), postural hypotension, degenerative joint disease, giddiness, and depression, the effects of certain medications on homeostasis, and/or environmental hazards or obstacles that interfere with safe mobility" [17].

5. Measurement of frailty in general practice

Frailty is recognized by a number of techniques as a clinical syndrome or phenotype (a group of symptoms that frequently co-occur to define a certain medical disease). Summative impairment lists and algorithms that are based on clinical judgment are typical of them. Frailty is defined by a number of factors, including physical inactivity and weight loss, gait speed, hand grip, visual impairment, fatigue, resistance, ambulation, as well as the inability to get up from a chair without using arms five times and a decreased energy level. Slow gait speed has been utilized alone as a frailty indicator despite its high correlation with functional decline and impairment. Presence of three or more of the five criteria like weight loss, tiredness, weak grip strength, slow walking speed, and low physical activity has been described as frailty phenotype is the most well-known and frequently used one originally defined by Fried et al. [2]. This phenotype was recently utilized to describe frailty as the most common condition causing death in community-dwelling older individuals. It has been validated as a predictor of unfavourable outcomes in major epidemiological investigations. The Fried et al. model is very strong since it recognizes frailty as a wasting condition and is clinically consistent and reproducible. On inpatient wards, however, a large number of very 'vulnerable' elderly patients are unable to take performance-based assessments and cannot be categorized by phenotypic measurements [3].

The fundamental benefit of Fried's approach is that it just calls for the evaluation of five factors: physical activity, grip strength, fatigue, and weight reduction [2]. Although this is reasonable in terms of primary care, there is a problem with the way the measure was put together. According to Fried's definition, frailty can be divided into three groups based on the total number of individual criteria that are met in each group (0: non-frail, 1 or 2: pre-frail, and 3, 4 or 5: frail). Retrospectively, using the lowest twentieth percentile criterion, individual criteria that are measured on a continuous scale (such as grip strength, walking speed, and physical activity) are dichotomized. There are also further stratifications. This calls for extensive statistical knowledge. Primary care physicians are not usually equipped with the necessary statistical knowledge or a reference sample, both of which are necessary for this. It is debatable if impairments of cognition and mood are left out of these models because frailty in the clinical world encompasses more than just weakness, slowness, and waste [4, 5].

Frailty can be measured as a multidimensional risk state that can be determined by the quantity rather than the type of health issues by seeing aging as the accumulation of impairments. The Frailty Index (FI) model develops an index as a percentage of deficits using a well-defined approach [13]. They have received strong validation in large, community-based research as a method of quantifying health state, with strong correlations to institutionalization, deteriorating disability, and death. A measure of frailty status can be obtained from data normally gathered during the examination of an older person because FIs can be created from various numbers and types of impairments. There are now studies looking into the clinical applicability and predictive validity of a FI produced from Comprehensive Geriatric Assessment.

6. Screening tools for frailty

One technique for detecting frailty is the Frailty Index (FI) which is a collection of health weaknesses, such as symptoms, signs, impairments, and diseases. The patient's FI score, which ranges from zero to one, is determined by the percentage of deficiencies present [18]. Different numbers and types of deficits may be employed in a FI with at least 30 deficits without significantly affecting the FI's features, allowing for use in and comparison of various datasets. Other frailty instruments, including the Tilburg Frailty Indicator, are more promising, according to other writers, who claim that the FI hasn't been validated in this context, is of limited utility due to its perceived complexity, and has only moderate discriminative power [19]. Others have asserted that the FI is a substantial predictor of unfavourable health outcomes, that it includes all crucial frailty indicators, that it is simple to calculate from regular administrative healthcare data, and that further research is needed to determine the FI's benefits in primary care [19].

7. Do we know how to detect and measure frailty?

At the turn of the century, a variety of models, explanations, and tools were put forth to operationalize the concept of frailty and identify those who were feeble. Two strategies were developed as a result of prospective, quantitative research on sizable samples of community-dwelling individuals; both strategies were presented in seminal publications released in 2001. The multisystem loss of physiological reserve that distinguishes frailty as a risk for a variety of unfavourable outcomes is referred to as the frailty phenotype and was first described by Fried et al. [20].

Fried's frailty phenotype may have a wide diffusion because it has a good face validity and only a few measurement-required factors. However, it has come under fire for limiting frailty to the physical components of health and ignoring mental health issues, which are common in old age and may heighten frailty, such as mood disorders or cognitive impairments [6]. But the five measures suggested by Fried et al. are probably also reflective of mental health: weariness is measured using items from a depression screening questionnaire, and new studies have shown links between frailty and cognitive impairments.

The "accumulation of deficits" concept, as defined by Mitnitski and Rockwood, is based on a frailty index that is calculated from numerous health-related indicators [11]. It alludes to the idea of advanced biological age in relation to the danger of passing away. The Canadian Study of Health and Aging data used in the development of this model included more than 90 distinct variables, including medical diagnoses, self-reported health issues or symptoms, physical manifestations, lab test outcomes, and functional challenges with ADLs. The frailty index, which is defined as their arithmetic total, is a variable-neutral measure. The selection of variables is based on three guiding principles: they point to health issues whose prevalence rises with age, they address multiple systems, and they do not reflect conditions that are always present in old age (and thus would not distinguish between people of the same chronological age). As long as there are enough factors included—at least 30 to 40—the set of variables chosen to compute the index of frailty may theoretically vary between different samples [13]. The "accumulation of deficits" hypothesis does not offer any hints as to the physiological processes producing frailty. But the wide variety of health deficiencies used to calculate the frailty index accommodate for the complexity of frailty, including its physical and psychological components.

All current frailty assessment tools were fundamentally validated by showing their potential correlation with unfavourable outcomes in population-based cohort studies. The frailty index generally predicts death better than the frailty phenotype. However, because it contains impairment indicators in its definition, it cannot be used to forecast the likelihood of functional deterioration.

The definition and validation of screening tools have received a lot of attention, but despite this, we still know very little about these two features outside of the frequently noted greater levels of frailty in women and in low socioeconomic groups [6, 15]. As a result, socioeconomic factors should be researched separately as susceptibility factors since they may interact with frailty to cause unfavourable health consequences. Early phases of frailty should be the most appropriate focus for intervention since they correspond to preclinical (or undetected) chronic diseases and functional decline and are more likely to be reversed.

The ability of frailty screening tools to properly predict negative outcomes at the individual level is still an open subject. These tools have been validated in population-based research and indicate prospective relationships with unfavourable outcomes. Frailty screening tools used in clinical practice to determine treatments must be specific and sensitive in order to avoid denying appropriate care to healthy individuals who are mistakenly labelled as pre-frail or frail [20]. The tools that are now in use often have excellent sensitivity but low specificity. Once age, sex, and chronic illnesses were taken into consideration in the population, it was discovered that a group of the most prevalent frailty markers had very little predictive value. Although it is appealing to use primary care data to quantify frailty, current evidence suggests that the frailty index is only weakly capable of forecasting unfavourable outcomes [21].

8. How we can prevent frailty?

The difference between an older person's chronological age and biologic age—and the requirement to treat older patients adequately by taking the second into account rather than the first—are at the core of geriatrics clinical practice. Although one or more chronic conditions are typically present in older patients, their number, combinations, severity, and impact on functional capacities are very diverse at any given age. As a result, although the prevalence of chronic diseases is highest in older age, chronological age does not always correspond to the risk of disability and death. An older person's fragility is frequently portrayed as a degree of inherent vulnerability. Although it tends to rise with age, it is unrelated to chronological age.

Many dependent older people are both frail and impaired because frailty can be the beginning of a developing dependency in activities of daily living (ADL). Frailty, however, does not always lead to old age infirmity, and not everyone who is fragile is always functionally dependent.

Although there are no known methods to reverse frailty, epidemiological research into the causes linked to its onset provide light on potential interventional methods. Because co-morbidities such cerebrovascular, chronic renal, and cardiovascular disease are linked to frailty, preventing these diseases early on may help to lower the prevalence of frailty in old life [22]. Quitting smoking in particular may offer advantages over simply preventing one disease. Smoking has been directly associated with the development of frailty because it is a potent inflammatory stimulation that brings on the inflow and activation of inflammatory cells. Despite the well-established link between inflammation and frailty, anti-inflammatory medications or foods with anti-inflammatory properties do not appear to be able to stop or delay the onset of frailty, according to observational and epidemiological research conducted to far [23].

Additionally, obesity and, in particular, the buildup of abdominal fat, are linked to greater frailty, as well as larger waist circumference are more likely to be fragile, as compared to older adults who are underweight [24]. Therefore, abdominal obesity in elderly individuals with low BMIs may be a new area of management. Physical activity may improve function without affecting weight loss due to decreased belly adiposity and enhanced oxidative activity [24]. Because they are sophisticated therapies that have the potential to change the accumulation of deficiencies across numerous systems, exercise, healthy eating, and improved education are of special interest as therapeutic methods for frailty. More research should be done to determine whether elderly patients who are frail would benefit from lengthier rehab stays in facilities that provide individualized exercise programs and nutritional assistance.

9. Prescribing in frail older people

The cost and quantity of prescription pharmaceuticals have increased as a result of the introduction of recommendations for the management of chronic diseases. The bioavailability of prescription drugs is impacted by altered pharmacokinetic responses that are related to frailty. Drug distribution is impacted by increases in body fat and decreases in lean body mass; low albumin levels diminish drug binding and hinder the activity of enzymes involved in drug metabolism [18]. Older persons also have pharmacodynamic changes that raise their risk of adverse drug reactions (ADRs), such as greater sensitivity to benzodiazepines and warfarin [19, 20].

Although co-morbidity or disability are not the same thing as frailty, many elderly persons who are frail have a number of chronic illnesses, functional impairment, and are given extensive prescription regimens. The drawbacks of polypill go beyond the dangers of taking individual medications. A greater chance of non-compliance and a noticeably increased risk of adverse drug reactions are linked to the use of more drugs. Regardless of the medication's reasons, older persons taking five or more drugs had a noticeably greater risk of delirium and falls. It has been demonstrated that when frailty is expressed as a co-morbidity index, ADRs rise in elderly people who are fragile. More research is needed to understand the independent impacts of frailty, although it is likely that a more robust person with a number of co-morbidities will tolerate ADRs better than a frailer person with a comparable list of co-morbidities. When prescribing drugs for elderly patients who are frail, goals of care should be carefully examined, even if the fundamental approach and concepts behind drug prescription should be identical for all patients. In people with short life expectancies, the hazards of secondary prevention can outweigh their advantages.

10. Are polypill necessary?

The shift in the elderly population's demographics poses a considerable challenges among physicians because older age is linked to a number of chronic ailments as hypertension, diabetes mellitus, arthritis, chronic heart disease, renal diseases, etc. Because of this, elderly people frequently take several drugs throughout the course of the day, a practice known as polypill. It can be characterized as the administration of more prescriptions than are clinically required and/or the usage of several medications, typically referred to as five or more prescribed drugs per day, which represents needless or undesirable drug use. Numerous research conducted worldwide have revealed that older persons often take 2–9 drugs each day. It was discovered that between 11.5 and 62.5% of older adults took improper medications [25].

Unfortunately, the signs and symptoms of polypill are typically demented and include: fatigue, sleepiness, or decreased alertness; constipation, diarrhoea, or incontinence; loss of appetite; confusion; falls; depression; or lack of interest in daily activities. They can also include: weakness; tremors; visual or auditory hallucinations; anxiety; or excitability; and/or dizziness.

In order to prevent any potential negative consequences, a patient who is older should have their polypill evaluated. To identify polypill and its negative effects, an interdisciplinary team should conduct a thorough medication review and risk assessment. Several tools, including Assess Review Minimize Optimize Reassess, Screening Tool to Alert Doctors to the Right Treatment, and Screening Tool to Older Person's Potentially Inappropriate Prescriptions, can be used to carry it out. Evaluation of the cause and effect of medication errors leading to ADRs is aided by the ADR probability scale and the Trigger tool for monitoring Adverse Drug Events in Nursing Homes. According to studies, Comprehensive Geriatric Assessment can help individuals take fewer prescriptions and daily medication doses overall.

The drug regimens of older people should be reviewed periodically in order to decrease the incidence and negative effects of polypill. If possible, a single agent or medication should be provided rather than a number of medications to address a particular condition. Where clinically warranted, medication dosages should be begun at a lower level and increased gradually as needed. Drugs that may be administered once or twice a day are preferable to those that must be administered three times a day. Drugs that are thought to be problematic should be stopped. If a medicine is used and neither a therapeutic benefit nor a clinical indication can be shown, the drug should be stopped. When many healthcare professionals prescribe the same medication for the same condition or disease, unnecessary medications should be discovered and removed. safer medications should drugs should be substituted with the higher risk medications.

Finding and avoiding polypill can assist elderly patients have better results and improve their quality of life. To prevent the negative consequences that polypill may have on an aged patient, medication review is crucial.

Increased risk of medication nonadherence, negative drug responses, drug interactions, and geriatric syndromes (falls, urine incontinence, cognitive impairment) are all consequences of polypill.

11. The prescription rules

1. Is it appropriate?

   Taking care of a new symptom as some symptoms (such as constipation—laxatives; vertigo—meclizine) appear to prompt a reflex prescription.
   However, take into account the following before beginning a medication:

2. Is something reversible?

   Dizziness brought on by a reduction in postural blood pressure so check for antihypertensive treatment, rather than starting new prescription for dizziness. Constipationmay be brought on by opioid analgesia, insist on any non-drug interventions (Example: increasing fibre to treat constipation). Before subjecting the patient to a number of medications, diagnosis must be confirmed, and disease-modifying therapies should not be withheld only to prevent polypill. Tight and meticulous treatment should not be considered to reduce disease-related mortality if the patient already has a short life expectancy (for example, cholesterol medicine in a patient with severe dementia or decreasing cholesterol and controlling blood sugar). The patient must be aware of the purpose of the treatment.

3. Do any conditions preclude its use where encounters likely to occur?

   Review the medication list and request information regarding the use of herbal and over-the-counter drugs. Computer prescribing, which automatically warns to potential concerns, is helpful in preventing drug-drug interactions.

4. What dosage should be started?

   Start low and go slow. Drug dosages are often better tolerated at lower doses and can be increased if there are no unfavourable side effects. For instance, 1.25 mg of ramipril is better than 10 mg with a postural drop in blood pressure when taking ACE inhibitors for heart failure. The benefits continue to rise as the dose is optimized.

5. How will the impact's evaluation be done?

   Plan a follow-up appointment and look for medication's effectiveness (e.g., has a dopamine agonist helped bradykinesia? Setting up precise therapy goals and carefully interviewing the patient and their family or carers are necessary when administering medication for less objective conditions (such as pain or cognition). When taking a statin, for example, check blood tests to determine effectiveness by lipid panel. Any negative side effects that the patient reports voluntarily, that are elicited by direct questions (such as a headache caused by dipyridamole), or that are necessary should be checked by blood tests (such as thyroid function while taking amiodarone). Side effects can be imperceptible and simple to miss. For instance, a patient with dementia may experience decreased hunger or attention for many different reasons. Even seemingly safe drugs like aspirin or iron can have an impact on hunger, and an antidepressant that was once successful can have a dulling effect on attention. A careful re-evaluation and a trial without the medicine are frequently beneficial.

6. Do not use it as a general rule.

   In geriatric medicine, a lot of prescribing is based on practical judgment and personally tailored assessments. There are always situations where it is necessary to break the rules in the best interests of the particular patient, even though most of what is detailed in the preceding pages is acceptable for most people.

Prescription cascades should be identified to prevent inappropriate polypill as shown in **Figure 2**.

First question should be thought of, "Is the patient reporting a symptom that could represent an adverse drug event?". Furthermore, "Is a new drug being considered to address an adverse event that may be related to a previously prescribed drug therapy?" "Could the initial drug be substituted for a safer alternative or could the dose be reduced, potentially eliminating the need for the subsequent drug therapy?". If so, "Does the patient need the initial drug therapy or could it be stopped?"

DOI: http://dx.doi.org/10.5772/intechopen.112464

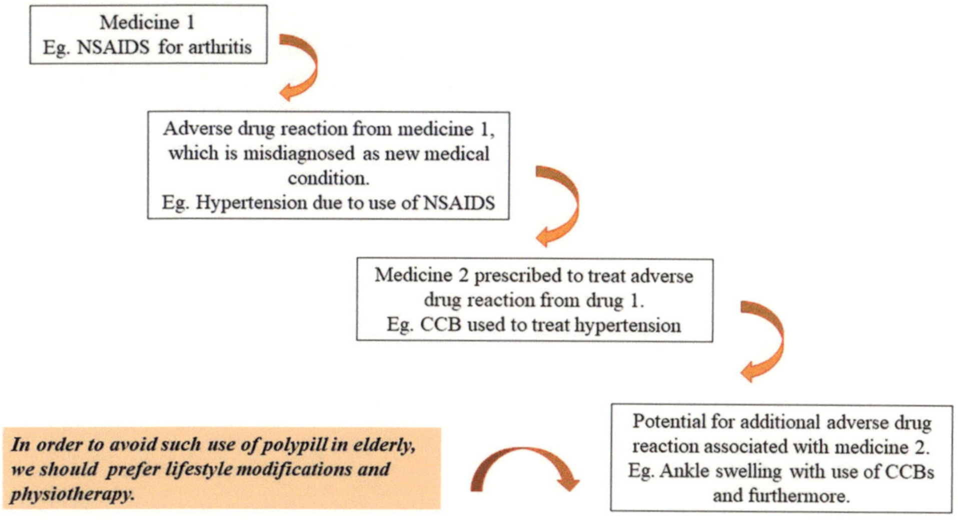

Figure 2.
Example of prescription cascade to avoid polypill. Non steriodal anti inflammatory drugs (NSAIDS), Calcium channel blockers (CCB).

Experience is necessary for this method, and the patient should always be monitored to determine how the decision affected them.

Although polypill has drawbacks, it is not universally viewed as a bad thing. It can also be harmful to deny individuals access to medicines because they are too old or already on too many medications.

Co-prescribing a medication to treat the anticipated bad impact may be justified when side effects are very probable but the treatment is unquestionably indicated, for instance: Opiates and laxatives, Steroids and bisphosphonates, An ACE inhibitor or furosemide together with a potassium-sparing diuretic, Nonsteroidal medications and a stomach-protecting substance.

Drug interactions for some diseases should be avoided since they are highly likely, but they may be tolerated for other diseases. For instance:

Although beta-blockers should not be used without caution in cases of asthma because of their positive effects on lowering cardiovascular risk, these warnings should not be taken as gospel. Since COPD frequently masquerades as "asthma" and has low beta-receptor responsiveness, cautious beta-blockade that is started in the hospital while keeping an eye on lung function may be suitable. Cardiovascular disease is common in diabetics, and the advantages of beta-blocker typically outweigh the risks. Although fludrocortisone (for postural blood pressure drop) will increase hypertension and produce ankle edema, it may be reasonable to accept the risk of hypertension if the postural drop is so severe that the patient is unable to move. If this is the best treatment option for a patient with chronic venous insufficiency, amlodipine may make their ankle edema worse.

12. Conclusion

Long life is not always equal to quality and good living, so focus should be on the health span, rather than the lifespan to decrease the burden of old age. WHO defines healthy aging as the "process of developing and maintaining the functional ability that enables wellbeing in oldage." Understanding the decline in functional ability of each biological system and identifying common biological targets and strategies based on the hallmarks of aging are key to delay in gage-associated decline. Identifying and avoiding the polypill can lead to better outcomes in the elderly patients and also helps in improving the quality of life by frequent prescription review to avoid adverse effects thence frailty.

Author details

Sunil Kumar and Nishtha Manuja*
Department of Internal Medicine, Datta Meghe Institute of Higher Education, Wardha, Maharashtra, India

*Address all correspondence to: nishtha_manuja@yahoo.in

References

[1] Fried LP, Tangen CM, Walston J, Newman AB, Hirsch C, Gottdiener J, et al. Frailty in older adults: Evidence for a phenotype. The Journals of Gerontology. Series A, Biological Sciences and Medical Sciences. 2001;**56**:M146-M156

[2] Kumar S. Frailty index – Assessment Tools in elderly: Feasibility in India. Annals of Geriatric Education and Medical Sciences. 2017;**4**(2):45-49.9

[3] Kumar S, Jain S, Wanjari A, Mandal S. Development and validation of a modified Frailty Risk Index as a predictor of mortality in rural elderly people. Asian Journal of Gerontology Geriatrics. 2019;**14**(1):15-22

[4] Ahmed N, Mandel R, Fain MJ. Frailty: An emerging geriatric syndrome. The American Journal of Medicine. 2007;**120**:748-753

[5] Hubbard RE, O'Mahony MS, Woodhouse KW. Characterising frailty in the clinical setting: A comparison of different approaches. Age and Ageing. 2009;**38**:115-119

[6] Abellan van Kan G, Rolland YM, Morley JE, Vellas B. Frailty: Toward a clinical definition. Journal of the American Medical Directors Association. 2008;**9**:71-72

[7] Rockwood K, Mitnitski A. Frailty defined by deficit accumulationand geriatric medicine defined by frailty. Clinics in Geriatric Medicine. 2011;**27**:17-26

[8] Bergman H, Ferrucci L, Guralnik J, et al. Frailty: An emerging research and clinical paradigm: Issues and controversies. The Journals of Gerontology. Series A, Biological Sciences and Medical Sciences. 2007;**62**:731-737

[9] Turner G, Clegg A, British Geriatrics Society; Age UK; Royal College of General Practioners. Best practice guidelines for the management of frailty: A British Geriatrics Society, Age UK and Royal College of General Practitioners report. Age Ageing. 2014;**43**:744-747

[10] Fillit H, Butler RN. The frailty identity crisis. Journal of American Geriatrics Society. 2009;**57**:348-352

[11] Clegg A, Bates C, Young J, et al. Development and validation of an electronic frailty index using routine primary care electronic health record data. Age and Ageing. 2016;**45**:353-360

[12] Searle SD, Mitnitski A, Gahbauer EA, Gill TM, Rockwood K. A standard procedure for creating a frailty index. BMC Geriatrics. 2008;**8**:24

[13] Kashikar Y, Nagarkar A. Prevalence and determinants of frailty in older adults in India. Indian Journal of Gerontology. 2016;**30**:364-381

[14] Hoogendijk EO, van der Horst HE, Deeg DJ, et al. The identification of frail older adults in primary care: Comparing the accuracy of five simple instruments. Age and Ageing. 2013;**42**:262-265

[15] Kulminski AM, Ukraintseva SV, Kulminskaya IV, Arbeev KG, Yashin AI. Cumulative deficits better characterize susceptibility to death in elderly people than phenotypic frailty: Lessons from the Cardiovascular Health Study. Journal of American Geriatric Society. 2008;**56**:898-903

[16] Rockwood K, Mitnitski A. Frailty in relation to the accumulation of deficits. The Journals of Gerontology. Series A, Biological Sciences and Medical Sciences. 2007;**62**:722-727

[17] Kumar S, Godhiwala P, Garikapati A, Jain S. Polypill therapy and frailty in elderly: Time to stop treating everything. Asian Journal of Medical Science. 2021;**12**(4):39-42

[18] Hilmer SN, Gnjidic D. The effects of polypill in older adults. Clinical Pharmacology and Therapeutics. 2009;**85**:86-88

[19] Linjakumpu T, Hartikainen S, Klaukka T, Veijola J, Kivelä SL, Isoaho R. Use of medications and polypill are increasing among the elderly. Journal of Clinical Epidemiology. 2002;**55**(8):809-817

[20] Rakesh KB, Chowta MN, Shenoy AK, Shastry R, Pai SB. Evaluation of polypill and appropriateness of prescription in geriatric patients: A crosssectional study at a tertiary care hospital. Indian Journal of Pharmacology. 2017;**49**:1620

[21] Maher RL, Hanlon J, Hajjar ER. Clinical consequences of polypill in elderly. Expert Opinion on Drug Safety. 2014;**13**:57-65

[22] Bonaga B, Sánchez-Jurado PM, Martínez-Reig M, Ariza G, Rodríguez-Mañas L, Gnjidic D, et al. Frailty, polypill, and health outcomes in older adults: The Frailty and Dependence in Albacete Study. Journal of the American Medical Directors Association. 2018;**19**:46-52

[23] Hasan SS, Kow CS, Verma RK, Ahmed SI, Mittal P, Chong DWK. An evaluation of medication appropriateness and frailty among residents of aged care homes in Malaysia: A cross-sectional study. Medicine. 2017;**96**:e7929

[24] Saum KU, Schottker B, Meid AD, Holleczek B, Haefeli WE, Hauer K, et al. Is polypill associated with frailty in older people? Results from the ESTHER cohort study. Journal of the American Geriatrics Society. 2017;**65**:e27-e32

[25] Thai M, Hilmer S, Pearson SA, Reeve E, Gnjidic D. Prevalence of potential and clinically relevant statin-drug interactions in frail and robust older inpatients. Drugs & Aging. 2015;**32**:849-856

Section 2

Fight against Obesity and Sedentary Lifestyle to Promote Health

Chapter 5

Sarcopenic Obesity: Focus on the Asian Population

Mukulesh Gupta and Tuhina Gupta

Abstract

Sarcopenic obesity (SO) is a condition observed in older adults, marked by a simultaneous presence of low muscle mass and high body fat mass. The document highlights the complex interplay of aging, hormonal changes, pro-inflammatory pathways, myocellular mechanisms, and oxidative stress as contributors to SO. It discusses the need for a standardized definition, as various criteria have been proposed over the years. The prevalence of SO varies in different populations, and its screening involves assessing body mass index (BMI) or waist circumference along with validated questionnaires. The document emphasizes the importance of accurate diagnostic methods, including measuring muscle mass, strength, and physical performance. The adverse health consequences of SO include increased risk of disability, cardiometabolic abnormalities, fractures, depression, mortality, and reduced quality of life. Lastly, the management of SO involves a multifaceted approach that focuses on gaining muscle mass while losing fat mass, primarily through resistance training, essential amino acid supplementation, dietary protein intake, and other emerging treatments.

Keywords: sarcopenic obesity, short physical performance battery (SPPB), appendicular lean mass, myosteatosis (MS), myofibrosis (MF)

1. Introduction

Normal aging is linked with 1% muscle loss from 30 years of age, which tends to accelerate after 70 years of age. In young adults, lean muscle mass, comprising around 50% of their overall bodyweight, declines to approximately 25% by the time they reach 75–80 years of age. After the age of 40, the rate of muscle loss can be as high as 8% per decade, and it increases to about 15% per decade after the age of 70. Individuals with diabetes experience a more significant reduction in muscle mass compared to others.

Hormones like total testosterone, which improves muscle protein synthesis, decrease by 1% per year, and the levels of dehydroepiandrosterone sulfate, a precursor to testosterone, also reduce with aging. Hyperthyroidism and chronic illness are also linked with muscle loss and reduced physical functioning. Sarcopenia was officially acknowledged as a medical condition in 2016 and was given a specific code in the International Classification of Diseases, tenth revision (ICD-10).

With age, apart from the development and progression of sarcopenia, the occurrence and prevalence of obesity also rise due to unhealthy diet and sedentary lifestyle [1]. The combination of high muscle mass and low fat mass is generally considered as healthy while the reverse as unhealthy. In obese individuals, metabolic change due to sedentary lifestyle, adipose tissue derangement, comorbidities, and so on can result in similar situation. A novel body composition category called sarcopenic obesity (SO) has emerged in recent times, characterized by the simultaneous presence of obesity and sarcopenia, encompassing both muscle mass and function [2]. This condition, also known as sarcopenic obesity, is gaining recognition as a clinical entity due to its substantial impact on patient-centered outcomes. It has multifactorial etiology, and its prevalence increases with age. SO is gaining attention because it is associated with many other age-related diseases that present as altered intercellular communication, dysregulated nutrient sensing, and mitochondrial dysfunction. Older adults identified with low muscle to fat ratio (MFR) have been found to have poor functional performance and high cardiometabolic risk. Higher cholecystectomy incidence is seen to be associated with low muscle mass, low muscle strength, sarcopenia, and sarcopenic obesity. Preliminary results suggest that SO may be associated with telomere shortening and may represent an important risk factor for accelerated aging than sarcopenia and obesity alone. Four body composition phenotypes have been proposed in older populations: normal, sarcopenic, obese, and sarcopenic obese. SO affects around 5–6% of Indian adults annually. SO is more common in older adults than in young adults. Both sarcopenia and obesity may individually cause threat for adverse health outcomes. But when combined, these two conditions can cause health threats that can be synergistically amplified. Studies have shown that SO is a better predictor of physical disability than sarcopenia or obesity alone.

The management of Sarcopenic Obesity involves implementing effective dietary and exercise strategies to counteract the negative outcomes. Additionally, there are various potential and developing treatments for SO, such as pharmacological interventions (including testosterone supplementation, selective androgen receptor modulators, myostatin inhibitors, and anti-obesity drugs), electrical acupuncture, whole-body electro-myo-stimulation, and the use of A2B agonists.

Conclusion: Sarcopenic obesity is emerging as a new and distinct category of obesity across the globe, which is clinically important. A theoretical methodological work (with a special focus on Asian population) aiming at providing practical-application guidelines is proposed.

2. Sarcopenic obesity (SO): an emerging challenge

Sarcopenic obesity is a new category of obesity in older adults who have high adiposity with low muscle mass. With aging, a progressive increase in fat mass, which normally peaks at about age 65 years in men and later in women, is observed. Aging is also associated with body fat distribution changes, visceral abdominal fat increase, and subcutaneous abdominal fat decrease. Moreover, in the elderly, ectopic fat deposition within non-adipose tissue such as the skeletal and cardiac muscle, liver, and pancreas has been observed. This phenomenon occurs even without significant changes in body mass index (BMI) or body weight. However, sarcopenia may arise in individuals with obesity at any age. The presence of obesity can cause a decline in muscle mass and function on its own, primarily because of the detrimental effects of metabolic disorders associated with adipose tissue. These disorders include oxidative stress, inflammation, insulin resistance, and a higher occurrence of chronic noncommunicable diseases.

2.1 Definition

BMI does not distinguish between fat mass and lean mass. In 2000, Baumgartner introduced the term of sarcopenic obesity (SO), a condition characterized by the coexistence of low muscle mass and a high body fat mass [3]. But it may underestimate sarcopenia in overweight and obese subjects, thus leading to an underdiagnosis of SO. Hence, more definitions of SO have been proposed.

In 2009, the European Working Group on Sarcopenia in Older People (EWGSOP) put forward a clinical definition of sarcopenia to facilitate its identification in older individuals. This definition suggested that sarcopenia should be diagnosed based on the simultaneous presence of two factors: low muscle mass and impaired muscle function, indicated by either low strength and/or low physical performance. The International Working Group on Sarcopenia proposed a similar definition in 2011, based on a low appendicular or whole-body fat-free mass combined with poor physical functioning [4]. In 2014, the Foundation for the National Institutes of Health Sarcopenia Project recommended defining sarcopenia using specific cut points for low lean mass (appendicular lean mass adjusted for BMI: 0.789 for men and 0.512 for women) and for muscle weakness (grip strength: 26 kg for men and 16 kg for women) [5]. However, to date, there is no universally accepted definition or classification for sarcopenia, or for sarcopenic obesity [6]. Studies have shown that SO is a better predictor of physical disability than sarcopenia or obesity alone. In 2022, European Society for Clinical Nutrition and Metabolism (ESPEN) and the European Association for the Study of Obesity (EASO) defined Sarcopenic obesity as the co-existence of obesity and sarcopenia (includes mass and function) [2].

2.2 Etiology and pathogenesis of SO

SO is a result of many complex interrelated mechanisms as mentioned below:

i. *Aging:* Many changes in body composition on aging due to lifestyle and reduced physical activity result in increased accumulation of fat, leading to SO phenotype.

ii. *Hormonal changes:* Hormonal changes that occur with aging result in insulin resistance, reduced thyroid hormone, increased cortisol levels, reduced growth hormones (GH), reduced insulin growth factor I (IGF-I), decreased sex steroids, and so forth, resulting in development of SO phenotype.

iii. *Pro-inflammatory pathways:* Aging results in increased levels of pro-inflammatory cytokines like TNF-α, IL-6, IL-1, and so forth. These inflammatory mediators cause muscle atrophy (increased catabolism) and adipocyte hypertrophy (infiltration of immune cells), both leading to SO.

iv. *Myocellular mechanisms:* One of the important parameter leading to SO is intramyocellular deposition of lipids (IMCLs), which promotes lipogenesis, inflammation, muscle insulin resistance, oxidative stress, and mitochondrial

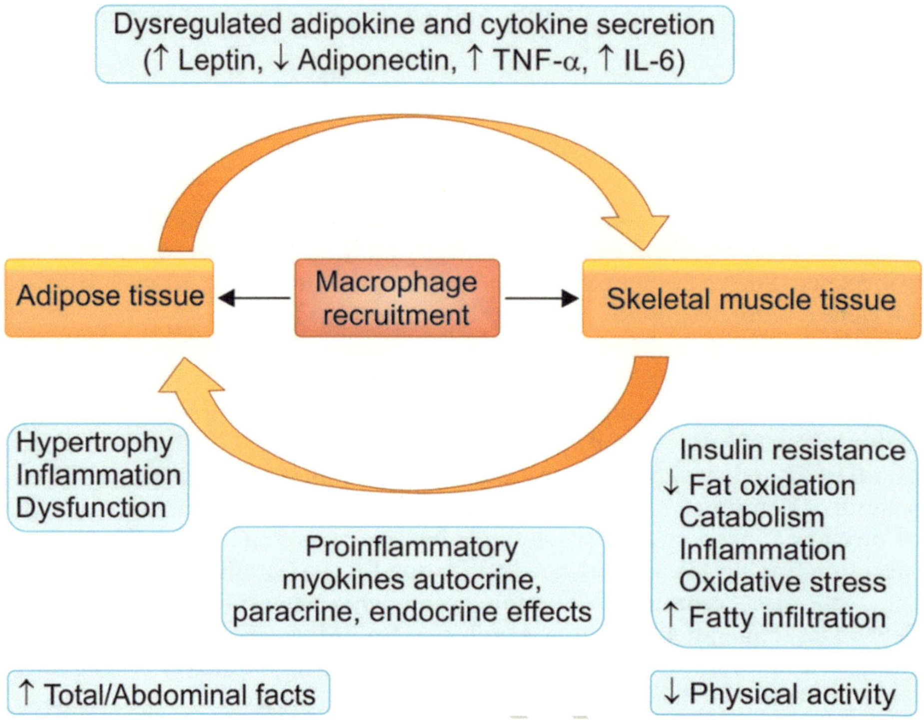

Figure 1.
Pathophysiology leading to Sarcopenic obesity.

dysfunction. This leads to impaired myocyte satellite cells differentiation/proliferation, leading to sarcopenia due to obesity.

v. *Oxidative stress:* Oxidative stress (OS) leads to an accumulation of ROS/RNS, accompanied by cellular damage. OS leads to infiltration of immune cells in the adipose tissue, leading to obesity and IR. OS also causes damage to the myocyte/satellite cells, leading to sarcopenia. Thus, OS can lead to sarcopenic obesity (**Figure 1**).

3. Sarcopenia in Asian populations: a distinct entity

Asian people have been seen to have lower muscle mass, weaker grip strength, slower gait speed, and greater body fat mass with central distribution; however, the intensity of age-associated muscle mass decline in the older Asian population remains comparatively unaltered, but the decline rate in muscle strength or physical performance with aging was more noteworthy. Additionally, Asian people showed greater elevation in fat mass and higher incidence of central obesity with aging, particularly in women.

3.1 Prevalence of sarcopenic obesity

The prevalence of sarcopenic obesity exhibits significant variation depending on the definitions used, assessment methods employed, and the specific populations under consideration.SO prevalence generally varies from 0 to 25% in older adults in different studies. The prevalence of sarcopenia in Indian population is approximately 39% [7]. A study conducted in Indian population in 2015 by ICMR concluded that the prevalence rate of obesity and central obesity varies from 11.8 to 31.3% and 16.9 to 36.3%, respectively [8]. SO affects around 5–6% of Indian adults annually.

4. Screening

It is based on concomitant presence of an elevated body mass index (BMI) or waist circumference (WC) with ethnicity specific cutoff points. Validated questionnaires, for example, SARC-F in older subjects [9]. The Asian Working Group for Sarcopenia (AWGS) recommends several preliminary screening methods for sarcopenia. These include measuring calf circumference (less than 34 cm in men and less than 33 cm in women), utilizing the SARC-F scale (≥4), or employing the SARC-Calf scale (≥11). During hospitalization, DXA or BIA can be used to enhance the accuracy of skeletal muscle mass (SMM) measurements (**Table 1**).

5. Diagnosis and method of assessment

According to the consensus of the Asian Working Group for Sarcopenia (AWGS) [11], the diagnosis of this ailment necessitates analysis of

a. Muscle mass

b. Muscle strength

c. Physical performance

5.1 Body composition

a. Dual-Energy X-ray Absorptiometry (DEXA),

b. Bioelectrical Impedance Analysis (BIA),

c. Ultrasound, computed tomography, and magnetic resonance imaging

In fact, both Dual Energy X-ray Absorptiometry (DXA) and Bioelectrical impedance analysis (BIA), the body composition methods which are usually recommended for definition of sarcopenia, are not able to recognize either myosteatosis (MS) or myofibrosis (MF) and also do not take into account muscle function in terms of strength and performance, and it is important because both muscle strength and performance decline quicker than muscle mass with aging.

To accurately diagnose SO, quantitative assessment of SMM and fat mass (FM) is vital. Computed Tomography (CT) and Magnetic Resonance Imaging (MRI) are considered as gold standard for accurate diagnosis of SMM and FM, but their use is limited due to high cost, limited availability, and radiation exposure in case of CT (**Table 2**).

SARC-F screen for sarcopenia: component question scoring

Strength: How much difficulty do you have in lifting and carrying 10 pounds?

- None 0
- Some 1
- A lot or unable 2

Assistance in walking: How much difficulty do you have walking across a room?

- None 0
- Some 1
- A lot, use aids, or unable 2

Rise from a chair: How much difficulty do you have transferring from a chair or bed?

- None 0
- Some 1
- A lot or unable without help 2

Climb stairs: How much difficulty do you have climbing a flight of 10 stairs?

- None 0
- Some 1
- A lot or unable 2

Falls: How many times have you fallen in the past year?

- None 0
- 1ess than 3 falls 1
- 4 or more falls 2

Data suggests that a SARC-F score of ≥4 best predicts the need for further, more comprehensive evaluation.

Table 1.
Validity of SARC-F Score: The SARC-F scale has demonstrated internal consistency and validity in identifying individuals at risk of experiencing negative outcomes associated with sarcopenia in various studies, including AAH, BLSA, and NHANES [10].

5.2 Skeletal muscle functional parameters

- Hand-grip strength (HGS),
- Knee extensor strength (adjusted for body mass in relevant populations),
- Chair-stand tests (5-time sit-to-stand test and the 30-second chair stand test)
- Gait speed test (GS) EWGSOP threshold <0.8 m/s
- Timed up and go (TUG)
- Short physical performance battery (SPPB)

Muscle functional cutoff points need to be validated as reference values for sex, ethnicity, and age stratum. Moreover, studies suggest the necessity to adjust hand-grip strength (HGS) to body mass.

Technique	Benefits	Limitations
Dual energy X-ray absorptiometry (DEXA)	Rapid Noninvasive Minimal radiation High precision Simultaneously measures SMM and FM	Portability Cost Limited access Dependent on patient hydration Does not distinguish between fat & lean mass
Computed axial tomography (CAT)	Identifies and quantifies myosteatosis High precision Differentiates between fat and lean mass	Portability Cost Limited access Radiation
Magnetic resonance imaging (MRI)	No radiation Identifies and quantifies myosteatosis High precision Differentiates between fat and lean mass	Portability Cost Limited access Long duration of test
Muscle tissue Ultrasound (US)	Low cost No radiation Real time imaging Inflammation and infiltration of muscle tissue can be differentiated	Dependent on type of ultrasound device and examiner's skill

Table 2.
Diagnosis techniques for Sarcopenic obesity.

5.3 Biomarkers for sarcopenia

Several Biomarkers have been studied. Irisin, a myokine that is released by skeletal muscles, is a potential biomarker for sarcopenia. Low irisin levels (<9.49 ng/mL) in T2DM patients is an independent risk factor for SO.

6. Staging

- *Stage-I*: No complications attributable to altered body composition and skeletal muscle functional parameters;

- *Stage-II*: Presence of at least one complication attributable to altered body composition and skeletal muscle functional parameters (e.g., metabolic diseases, disabilities resulting from high FM and-or low muscle mass, and cardiovascular and respiratory diseases).

7. Adverse health consequences of SO

7.1 SO has been associated with major clinical implications

Increased risk of disability, mobility limitations, and overall impaired physical capacity; elevated risk of cardiometabolic abnormalities such as insulin resistance, dyslipidaemia, hypertension, type 2 diabetes, and low-grade inflammation; increased risk of fractures; depression and compromised overall psychological health; poor outcomes in cancer; increased mortality risk; reduced health-related quality of life;

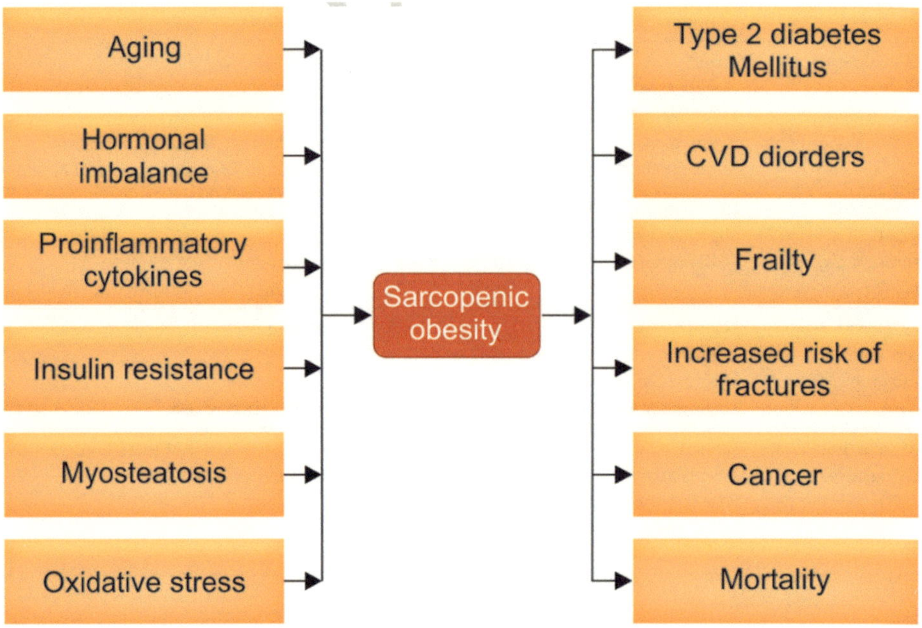

Figure 2.
Sarcopenic obesity: causes and consequences (CVD: cardiovascular disease).

and institutionalization and expanded healthcare costs. However, the cross-sectional design of related studies fails to provide solid information on causal relationships. This highlights the need for longitudinal studies to elucidate the real impact of SO on the onset and progression of specific diseases (**Figure 2**).

8. Management of sarcopenic obesity

Two approaches need to be pursued at the same time:

Gaining SMM while losing FM: The effects of any intervention should focus on changes in body composition and functional parameters and not be measured as changes of body weight alone. If the treatment strategy is limited to only weight loss interventions, there can be inevitable health risks for elderly individuals, mainly related to the concomitant loss of bone and skeletal muscle mass and exacerbation of osteosarcopenia [12].

Therefore, it is very important to focus on body fat loss and maintenance or accretion of muscle mass, so as to maintain strength, function, and resting metabolic rate (RMR). Combined therapy of nutrition along with exercise is the most accepted strategy for these goals [13].

8.1 Resistance training

Resistance training is one the most accepted training for older adults that can improve body composition without weight loss.

Fiatarone and colleagues showed that an eight-week training program of resistance training led to an increase in muscle mass in even frail, institutionalized 90-year-old men and women [14]. Weight training (resistance training) for three days a week increases muscle mass, with a decrease in fat mass in healthy men and women aged 50–75 years, with body weight remaining unchanged [15].

Resistance training also induces changes in muscle fiber in healthy men and women aged 60 years or older.

Along with severe calorie restriction, resistance training is beneficial. Calorie restriction usually leads to a reduction in both fat and lean mass. Resistance exercise, when prescribed along with calorie restriction, can help prevent muscle loss. As a result, this can lead to a decrease in fat mass along with maintaining muscle mass.

8.2 Essential amino acids (EAA) supplementation

EAA supplementation along with resistance exercise can enhance muscle protein synthesis and can improve body composition by increasing lean mass, not fat mass [16]. In men and women aged 25–35 years, ingestion of essential amino acids before intense resistance exercise resulted in significant increase in muscle protein synthesis and an increase in lean mass [17]. Similarly, 12 weeks of resistance training with the consumption of protein supplement (17 g of essential amino acids) twice a day by healthy young men stimulated greater gain in lean mass compared with resistance training alone [18]. Administration of 15 g of essential amino acids to healthy middle-aged men, along with resistance training program, resulted in attenuation of loss of muscle and gains in fat.

8.3 Dietary protein

Even without resistance exercise, a high protein diet may itself provide an anabolic environment for promoting retention or accretion of muscles over time. A study conducted by Solerte and colleagues concluded that in older men and women aged 64–84 years with sarcopenia, oral supplementation with 16 g per day of essential amino acids was sufficient to increase lean mass in 8 months [19]. This effect persisted over time and resulted in a decrease in TNFα, which is found to be elevated in sarcopenic process. Protein supplementation also prevents muscle loss during calorie restriction, with minimal energy deficit. Higher consumption of high-quality protein (aiming for 1–1.2 g/kg/d or even higher intake 1.2–1.5 g/kg/d) than the current RDA might be advantageous for older adults and malnourished medical in patients [20]. It is also seen that when an individual consumes insufficient diet, the loss of protein can be lessened or even stopped by the addition of carbohydrates or fats to the food and is regarded as the "protein-sparing action" of carbohydrates and fats.

8.4 Treatment strategies

See **Table 3**.

8.5 Newer emerging treatments

Electrical acupuncture and whole-body electro-myo-stimulation, in conjunction with nutritional supplementation, are emerging and effective approaches to bring about alterations in body composition. Whole body vibration therapy has also found to be a safe and convenient technique to cause neuromuscular activation and simulate the contraction of skeletal muscle. A recent study has demonstrated that the adenosine A2B receptor (A2B) is highly expressed in muscle tissue and brown adipose tissue (BAT) and may be a target for SO.

Treatment modality	Mechanism	Comments
Testosterone and Selective androgen receptor modulators (SARM)	Increase muscle mass by increasing IGF-1 decreasing inflammatory markers	Conflicting results Early studies showed good results in cancer patients
Myostatin inhibitors	Enhance skeletal muscle growth. Inhibiting SMM loss	Promising results in cancer related SMM loss
Mesenchymal stem cells	Precursors for skeletal muscle tissue	Promising result as an early treatment for sarcopenia Cost, regulatory, and ethical constraints.
Anamorelin (oral ghrelin analogue)	Anabolic effects Anti-inflammatory properties	Safe, well tolerated in cancer patients with cachexia
Anti-obesity medications	Promote weight loss. Minimal effects on SMM	Approved for non-geriatric population Not known in older adults
Bariatric surgery	Results in weight loss	Unknown safety and efficacy in older patients May exacerbate weight loss-induced sarcopenia and osteoporosis
Neuromuscular activation	Enhances muscle contraction efficiency and functions	Mixed data on efficacy and safety

Table 3.
Novel treatment strategies.

9. Unmet needs, challenges, and knowledge gaps

- To establish a robust and standardized definition of SO.
- To establish reliable techniques to assess body composition for diagnosing SO.
- Further elucidate on descriptive epidemiology of SO, beyond weight loss, morbidity, and mortality, focusing more on patient-centric outcomes like physical functionality and quality of life.
- At present, no specific dietary plans have been tested in populations suffering from SO. Several aspects like the type of protein, optimal concentration of amino acids to be given, and specificity of the amino acids needs to be established.
- To acquire more knowledge regarding optimal frequency, duration, and intensity of exercise (aerobic and resistance). Also, to evaluate if diet and exercise can be combined with pharmacotherapies such as testosterone supplements.

10. Conclusions and future directions

The convergence of two conditions – a growing aging population and increasing obesity rates – has led to an increase in the prevalence of SO, which is defined as the concurrent presence of sarcopenia and obesity in the same individual. SO can lead to an increase in risk of disability, CV disorders, hospitalization, and impaired quality of life and mortality. Because of such negative effects of SO, its effective diagnosis, prevention, and treatment emerge as a top priority among researchers and clinicians.

Sarcopenic obesity (SO) carries significant implications for public health, as it is connected to frailty, falls, disability, and heightened risks of morbidity and mortality.

The thin fat Indian phenotype, characterized by higher body fat composition and lower muscle mass (sarcopenia), makes individuals of Asian Indian descent more susceptible to muscle loss and metabolic disorders. Compared to their white or African counterparts. The rising prevalence of this condition among younger populations is a cause for concern.

To further advance the current knowledge, the scientific community should try to establish a robust definition and a reliable assessment/diagnostic method, conduct more patient-centric trials, and, finally, obtain concluding evidences with the help of trials for dietary and resistance training interventions.

Author details

Mukulesh Gupta[1*] and Tuhina Gupta[2]

1 Udyan Health Care Pvt Ltd, Lucknow, UP, India

2 SGT Medical College and Hospital, Gurgaon, India

*Address all correspondence to: drmukulesh@yahoo.com

References

[1] Ciudin A, Simó-Servat A, Palmas F, Barahona MJ. Sarcopenic obesity: A new challenge in the clinical practice. Endocrinología, Diabetes y Nutrición (English ed.). 2020;**67**(10):672-681

[2] Donini LM, Busetto L, et al. Definition and diagnostic criteria for sarcopenic obesity: ESPEN and EASO consensus statement. Clinical Nutrition. 2022;**41**:990-1000

[3] Baumgartner RN. Body composition in healthy aging. Annals of the New York Academy of Sciences. 2000;**904**(1):437-448

[4] Fielding RA, Vellas B, Evans WJ, Bhasin S, Morley JE, Newman AB, et al. Sarcopenia: An undiagnosed condition in older adults. Current consensus definition: Prevalence, etiology, and consequences. International working group on sarcopenia. Journal of the American Medical Directors Association. 2011;**12**(4):249-256

[5] Studenski SA, Peters KW, Alley DE, Cawthon PM, McLean RR, Harris TB, et al. The FNIH sarcopenia project: Rationale, study description, conference recommendations, and final estimates. Journals of Gerontology Series A: Biomedical Sciences and Medical Sciences. 2014;**69**(5):547-558

[6] Cruz-Jentoft AJ. European working group on sarcopenia in older people: Sarcopenia: European consensus on definition and diagnosis. Report of the European working group on sarcopenia in older people. Age and Ageing. 2010;**39**:412-423

[7] Rahman R, Wilson BP, Paul TV, Yadav B, Kango Gopal G, Viggeswarpu S. Prevalence and factors contributing to primary sarcopenia in relatively healthy older Indians attending the outpatient department in a tertiary care hospital: A cross-sectional study. Aging Medicine. 2021;**4**(4):257-265

[8] Ahirwar R, Mondal PR. Prevalence of obesity in India: A systematic review. Diabetes & Metabolic Syndrome: Clinical Research & Reviews. 2019;**13**(1):318-321

[9] Malmstrom TK, Morley JE. SARC-F: A simple questionnaire to rapidly diagnose sarcopenia. Journal of the American Medical Directors Association. 2013;**14**(8):531-532

[10] Malmstrom TK, Miller DK, Simonsick EM, Ferrucci L, Morley JE. SARC-F: Aa symptom score to predict persons with sarcopenia at risk for poor functional outcomes. Journal of Cachexia, Sarcopenia and Muscle. 2016;**7**(1):28-36.Available from: https://pubmed.ncbi.nlm.nih.gov/27066316/

[11] Limpawattana P, Assantachai P, Krairit O, Kengkijkosol T, Wittayakom W, Pimporm J, et al. The predictors of skeletal muscle mass among young Thai adults: A study in the rural area of Thailand. Biomedical Research (India). 2016;**27**(1):29-33

[12] Koliaki C, Liatis S, Dalamaga M, Kokkinos A. Sarcopenic obesity: Epidemiologic evidence, pathophysiology, and therapeutic perspectives. Current Obesity Reports. 2019;**8**(4):458-471

[13] Benton MJ, Whyte MD, Dyal BW. Sarcopenic obesity: Strategies for management. AJN The American Journal of Nursing. 2011;**111**(12):38-44

[14] Fiatarone MA, Marks EC, Ryan ND, Meredith CN, Lipsitz LA, Evans WJ. High-intensity strength training in nonagenarians: Effects on skeletal muscle. Journal of the American Medical Association. 1990;**263**(22):3029-3034

[15] Kerksick C, Thomas A, Campbell B, Taylor L, Wilborn C, Marcello B, et al. Effects of a popular exercise and weight loss program on weight loss, body composition, energy expenditure and health in obese women. Nutrition & Mtabolism. 2009;**6**(1):1-7

[16] Kerksick CM, Arent S, Schoenfeld BJ, Stout JR, Campbell B, Wilborn CD, et al. International Society of Sports Nutrition position stand: Nutrient timing. Journal of the International Society of Sports Nutrition. 2017;**14**(1):33

[17] Esmarck B, Andersen JL, Olsen S, Richter EA, Mizuno M, Kjaer M. Timing of postexercise protein intake is important for muscle hypertrophy with resistance training in elderly humans. The Journal of Physiology. 2001;**535**(1):301-311

[18] Kraemer WJ, Hatfield DL, Volek JS, Fragala MS, Vingren JL, Anderson JM, et al. Effects of amino acids supplement on physiological adaptations to resistance training. Medicine & Science in Sports & Exercise. 2009;**41**(5):1111-1121

[19] Solerte SB, Gazzaruso C, Bonacasa R, Rondanelli M, Zamboni M, Basso C, et al. Nutritional supplements with oral amino acid mixtures increases whole-body lean mass and insulin sensitivity in elderly subjects with sarcopenia. The American Journal of Cardiology. 2008;**101**(11):S69-S77

[20] Deer RR, Volpi E. Protein intake and muscle function in older adults. Current Opinion in Clinical Nutrition and Metabolic Care. 2015;**18**(3):248

Chapter 6

Movement and Aging

Emilia Patricia Zarco, Anne Gibbone and Hanna Matatyaho

Abstract

Movement is a fundamental function of life. Human beings move through the act of breathing before they learn language and speak. Movement is central to all of life's processes: growth and development, energy production and utilization, and environmental adaptation. This chapter will explore the power of human movement and how it can be harnessed to address the challenges of aging. Movement in this chapter refers to physical activity and exercise. The challenge of aging for the future is not simply prolonging human life at any cost or by any means but rather extending self-sufficiency and quality of life. Aging adults need to keep on moving to keep their independence, self-care and improve their quality of life. The chapter will present current knowledge and new insights from contemporary research as we explore how physical activity and exercise can help address challenges of aging in these areas: musculoskeletal health, pain, immune system and brain health.

Keywords: movement, physical activity, exercise, health promotion, aging

1. Introduction

Movement comes from the word "movere" which means to move. It is the act or process of moving. In a broader perspective, it is change or development. This chapter will focus on physical activity and exercise as movement. The World Health Organization (WHO) defines physical activity as any bodily movement that is produced by the contraction of skeletal muscle and that increases energy expenditure above a basal level. It refers to all movements including during leisure time, for transport to get to and from places or as part of a person's work. The US Centers for Disease Control and Prevention (CDC) also defines exercise as a form of physical activity that involves planned, structured and repetitive bodily movement with the goal of improving or maintaining health or fitness. Although all exercise is physical activity, not all physical activity is exercise.

The challenge of aging for the future is not simply prolonging human life at any cost or by any means but rather extending self-sufficiency and quality of life [1]. Movement is critical to address the changes of aging that prevent self-sufficiency and affect quality of life. Physical activity is required for self-care and determines an individual's level of independence or self-sufficiency. This challenge is compounded by the fact that 1.4 billion adults (27.5% of the world's adult population) or more than 1 in 4 adults do not meet the recommended level of physical activity to improve and protect their health [2]. Furthermore, both men and women become less active as they get older despite clear evidence that being active benefits older adults in relation

 IntechOpen

to preventing falls, remaining independent, reducing isolation and maintaining social links to improve psychosocial health [2].

The cost of physical inactivity is not only chronic diseases and premature deaths but a large economic burden. The WHO global status report on physical activity in 2022 states that physical inactivity costs health care systems US$ 27 billion a year due to preventable non-communicable diseases (NCDs). In the US, half of all American adults have one or more preventable chronic diseases like obesity, type 2 diabetes, heart disease, many types of cancer, depression, anxiety and dementia resulting in approximately $117 billion in annual health care costs and about 10 percent of premature mortality [3]. Furthermore, WHO projects almost 500 million (499,208 million) new cases of preventable NCDs between the years 2020–2030 if there is no change in the current prevalence of physical inactivity. The burden of new cases is highest among lower income countries (41 percent), with the Western Pacific Region predicted to be hardest hit. Globally, hypertension (47% prevalence accounting 22% health care cost), depression (43% accounting 28% health care cost) leads new cases of preventable NCDs. Dementia will account for 21% of health care costs due to the nature of its management and duration for which it is needed.

To explore how movement through increasing physical activity levels and engaging in regular exercise will help address aging challenges, a narrative review of relating movement with the four areas of health were chosen as the focus of the literature search: musculoskeletal health, pain, immune system and brain health. From the authors' discussion, these are the health areas that movement will impact directly or indirectly and will influence the aging populations' independence, self-sufficiency and quality of life. A preliminary search to validate the idea of relating aging with the four areas was conducted in the ONEsearch database. The key words "aging" paired with each of the areas of focus: musculoskeletal health, pain, immune system and brain health was used, and only peer-reviewed articles were included. The inclusion and exclusion criteria were formulated and refined after the preliminary search. The inclusion criteria included the following: worldwide peer-reviewed articles from 2020 and onward, English publications only, all types of research (quantitative and qualitative primary and secondary studies and tertiary research) were considered, and no dissertation work was included.

The evidence about the health benefits of regular physical activity is well established supported by studies that examined the role of physical activity in health and disease. There is evidence that even lower intensity activities demonstrate cardiometabolic and health benefits in an aging population [4]. A systematic review [13] found that 2.5 hour/week (equivalent to 30 min daily of moderate intensity activity on 5 days a week) compared with no activity was associated with a reduction in mortality risk of 19%, while 7 hour/week of moderate activity compared with no activity reduced the mortality risk by 24%. [5]. These studies clearly emphasize the importance of avoiding inactivity to delay death from all causes.

As one ages, being self-sufficient and pain free are among the utmost desires in sustaining a high quality of life [6]. Knowledge and practices that have been proven to regulate those goals have and continue to lead directly to movement [1]. Movement is dynamic and changes throughout the lifespan due to changes in musculoskeletal or nervous systems, fatigue, posture, injury, disease, or the environment. Changes related to age, include but are not limited to, changes in muscle fiber type, reduced vision, balance, range of motion, base of support, strength, reaction time and vestibular function in addition to increased postural sway, flexed posture, and pain. These changes influence functional mobility, balance and posture in older adulthood.

However, it is important to emphasize that these changes are controllable through movement training and exercise.

2. Movement and musculoskeletal health

Musculoskeletal deficits are among the most detrimental effects of aging due to loss of muscular strength, flexibility, balance and functional ability [7]. Loss of muscle strength accelerates with age. By the age of 75–85 years, a typical person has lost about 45–50% of their muscle strength and by the age of 85, more than 55% [1]. Muscle strength plays a role in walking speed as weak muscles provide less power to support walking speed. Regular strength and neuromuscular training assists in reversing or slowing down a decline in walking speed due to the aging process. Joints are subject to the state of muscles, connective tissue and cartilage and concentrating on stretching and ROM exercises will aid in improving flexibility in older adults.

Sarcopenia, the loss of muscle mass, strength and function affects 10–50% of people over 60 years of age [8]. It is considered a precursor syndrome for the physical manifestation of frailty leading to impaired mobility and reduced independence. It has been shown that older adults with sarcopenia have poorer bone health [9]. Over time osteoblast activity is reduced affecting bone loss and skeletal strength. Older adults engaging in high physical activity/low sedentary behaviors have greater skeletal muscle strength and muscle power [10]. Resistance training exercise helps to maintain muscle strength and size in older years. Inactive adults after the age of 60 have less strength due to sarcopenia or loss of muscle mass and exercise clearly helps to maintain muscle mass needed for daily living activities and injury prevention [11]. Exercise, proper diet and endocrinological balance are recommended as interventions that are interconnected to improve musculoskeletal health and quality of life.

Obesity, which is involved in the development of many chronic diseases, also affects musculoskeletal health. Older adults with a BMI of 30 kg/m2 or greater significantly demonstrate functional limitations [12]. Being overweight and/or obese has been suggested to lead to alterations in the musculoskeletal system that place overweight individuals at higher risk of musculoskeletal pain and restricted range of movement [13]. There is a dose-response relationship between obesity and knee osteoarthritis (OA), meaning the greater an individual's BMI, the greater the likelihood of developing OA [14]. Furthermore, obese adults with BMI over 35 perform poorly on tasks of executive function involving planning and mental flexibility when compared to normal individuals [15]. Older obese adult males showed deficits in cognitive functioning when completing cognitive tasks evaluating learning and visual memory [16]. The multidimensional nature of mobility issues among older adults with obesity requires a multidisciplinary approach to assessment and intervention with movement training (e.g., postural control and motor planning) as requirements.

Activities of daily living (ADL's) are used as a gauge of functional independence. Physical activity improves physical function among individuals of all ages, enabling them to conduct their daily lives with energy and without undue fatigue. This is true for older adults, for whom improved physical function reduces risk of falls and fall-related injuries and contributes to their ability to maintain independence. Among the elderly, fall-related injuries are a primary public health challenge [2]. Furthermore, projections of fall-related injuries continue to increase [17, 18]. Aging consequently worsens the efficacy of musculoskeletal systems and functional abilities [7]. Due to the increasing frequency of falls among the vastly growing population of older adults, targeted interventions to minimize fall risks are of utmost priority. Physical activity in general for the elderly has proven reductions in the rate of fall related injuries [19, 20]. However, correlating specific activity programs is challenging given the vast array of types of exercises, individual differences and limitations of high-quality clinical trials. Programs that focus on balance [21] and have high doses of physical activity have been proven successful in fall reduction [20]. Increased reaction time as one ages is a proven risk factor in falls [22]. Similarly changes in gait and mobility from aging are associated with functional decline [23] and gait kinematics have been linked to predicting fall risk [24–26]. Older adults exhibit several changes in gait and paired with increased reaction time and decreased strength, endurance and visual acuity, falls are a major public health issue. Identifying training programs that focus on decreasing the risk of falls are of tremendous value. Although neurophysiological changes as one ages will occur, reaction and response time reduction is curtailed by regular physical activity.

Functional mobility, which requires both strength and flexibility, is another musculoskeletal challenge among older adults. Regular physical activity, specifically stretching, has been shown to create instantaneous and long-lasting changes to maximal joint range of motion and improves flexibility and functional mobility. Several studies reported that stretching efficacy was not limited to the targeted joint being moved [27–29]. For example, unilateral stretching performed on one lower limb also increased the range of motion of the contralateral limb; stretching of the lower limb increased the maximal range of motion of the distant upper limbs and vice versa. The role of fascia and connective tissues provides an explanation of the efficacy of stretching beyond the targeted joint. Recent histologic findings showed that fascia contains contractile cells, free nerve endings, and mechanoreceptors and therefore plays a proprioceptive and mechanically active role that functions as a body-wide mechanosensitive signaling network [30]. Full body exercises that include full body stretching therefore offer more benefits for musculoskeletal health.

3. Movement and pain

As we age, pain is viewed as an inevitable part of life. Low back pain, for example, is one of the most common and complex musculoskeletal ailments. Reducing low back pain in many cases may be accomplished through improving strength, balance and flexibility. We begin with little aches and pains due to sports injuries, to more extreme injuries due to falls. In order to address pain, we begin by taking over the counter medication to numb the pain, but persistent pain sometimes occurs. In most cases, over-the-counter medication helps, and we continue with our daily living activities. According to the Consumer Healthcare Product Association (2023) approximately 23% of U.S. adults use Acetaminophen weekly. The Mayo Clinic (2023) states that Acetaminophen is "usually recommended as the first line treatment for mild to moderate pain." The struggle to manage pain is rather complex and has been discussed with much detail in the last decade, but pain management has been an integral part of medicine throughout history, where medication was almost always the preferred choice. In the 17th Century European doctors gave opium to their patients to relieve pain and by the 20th Century morphine and heroin were used to control pain [31]. While opioid use can be very effective in pain management relief, The American Society of Anesthesiologists states that it is also highly addictive. In fact, they report that "The risk of addiction is especially high when opioids are used to manage chronic pain over a long period of time" [32]. Older adults should be given the lowest analgesic dose for the shortest possible time to adequately manage their pain.

But what is pain? Pain, as described by the International Association for the Study of Pain (IASP) is, "an unpleasant sensory and emotional experience associated with, actual or potential tissue damage, or described in terms of such damage" [33]. There are two major types of pain: acute pain and chronic pain. Acute pain comes on quickly, can be severe, but in most cases a temporary condition that does not last for a long period of time. Chronic pain lasts beyond normal tissue healing time, generally taken to be 12 weeks/3 months and limits quality of life because it contributes to disability, anxiety, depression, sleep disturbances, poor quality of life and healthcare costs [34].

Pain among older adults leads to functional impairment, sleep disturbance, reduced socialization, depression, reduced mobility and impaired or slowed rehabilitation. There is an estimated 70–80% reduction in the ability to perform activities of daily living among older adults with pain. They also exhibit decreased gait speed, weaker grip strength and decreased self-reported physical activity [35]. Frailty, a common clinical syndrome among older adults often display reduced functional reserve and pain related impairments profoundly impact cognition and independence [36]. Pain is the most common reason people seek health care and the leading cause of disability in the world. In 2011, one in every five adults worldwide suffers from pain and one in every 10 adults is diagnosed with chronic pain each year [37]. The 2020 Global Pain Index reports that one third of the world's population is in pain everyday [38]. Acute pain is experienced regularly by up to 49–83%of elderly individuals above the age of 60 living in care homes and 40% of elderly individuals living in the community [38]. The prevalence of chronic pain among US adults ranged at 20.5–21.8% [39]. According to the Center for Practical Bioethics (2021) more than 116 million Americans are impacted by chronic pain, resulting in high healthcare costs. A report published by John Elflein [40] who conducted a survey in 2021 with 29,482 participants over the age of 18, showed that 26.8% of adults between the ages of 45 and 64; 30% of adults between the ages of 65 and 84; and 34.3% of adults 85 and over live with chronic pain in the United States. Chronic pain, especially in the elderly population, is more prevalent as pain is a frequent side effect of chronic illness. Although the aforementioned study did not discuss the causes of pain, it did demonstrate that chronic pain increases with age. While each individual's level and frequency of pain differs, as one ages, the duration of pain increases [41]. Stressful situations, depression and anxiety can exacerbate chronic pain because pain and these mental health states share overlapping nerve biological pain pathways in the brain. Prevalence of pain is common among the older age group highlighting the need for pain management that goes beyond analgesics and considering alternative options [42].

For many years, the non-pharmacological treatment choice for pain included recommendations for rest and inactivity [34]. However, movement or physical activity programs and exercise regimens are increasingly promoted to reduce chronic pain and improve mental health and physical functioning. Although pain is a normal protective response to injury and potentially harmful stimuli, prolonged or dysfunctional neuromuscular adaptations in response to pain may contribute to disability and chronicity in a variety of pain conditions [43]. Clinically, pain produces a large range of motor adaptations. This ranges from subtle motor compensations during task completion to complete avoidance of painful movements and/or activities [44]. Movement, individualized exercise programs and specific motor learning/functional tasks are often prescribed to help decrease pain and restore/improve function.

Studies provide evidence of the effectiveness of exercise for the treatment of pain. For example, exercise is effective for the management of chronic low back pain and for fibromyalgia strength, endurance training and stretching of the neck and upper extremities improve neck pain [45].

Physical therapy or physiotherapy is another non-pharmacological treatment for pain. Physical therapists or physiotherapists are considered movement experts who treat pain and improve quality of life through hands-on approaches: stretching, soft tissue release, joint mobilizations, fascial release, etc. Treatment also includes exercise-based approaches to strengthen muscles, improve balance and sharpen coordination. Physical therapy takes on a more holistic approach to pain relief because the interventions are based in the knowledge that all forces in the body affect each other. It works to restore the balance of coordination, flexibility and strength so that movement, blood flow and nerve functioning are facilitated. For example, pain due to a nerve pinch may happen because of compression from a muscle or fascia. Reducing the strain and restoring fluid movement through physiotherapy helps alleviate the pain. Many of the exercises used in a physical therapy session are encouraged to continue at home. Physical therapy works to restore movement and improve functional mobility, eliminate pain and reduce the need for surgery and pain medicines like opioids.

Studies also support that those engaging in regular physical activity are associated with less frequent back pain and reduced incidence of musculoskeletal pain [46, 47]. Some studies show that regular physical activity may reduce pain sensitivity, and some demonstrate no change, but greater pain sensitivity has never been observed. It should be noted that some acute exacerbation of chronic pain when beginning an exercise program may happen and therefore the need to gradually increase physical activity is critical with the goal of eventually reaching recommended guidelines. Regular exercise leads to chronic adaptations that provide the greatest benefit to addressing pain. It is recommended that engaging in physical activity at a young age builds muscle, helps with range of motion, and improves overall movement.

4. Movement and the immune system

As we grow older, our immune system slows down, weakens, and loses the ability to fight against illness, such as infections, cancer, and appropriate wound healing [48]. Our immune system plays an important role in protecting us from harmful substances, germs, and cell changes. It is made up of two parts: the innate immune system and the adaptive immune system. Innate immunity responds immediately to an invading pathogen, is antigen-independent, and has no immunologic memory [49]. Innate immunity is known as the first line of defense against germs or foreign substances. Adaptive immunity is antigen-dependent and antigen-specific and has immunologic memory which enables for an immune response when it recognizes the same antigen [49]. Inflammation is the body's immune response to any form of irritant.

A review conducted by Ghauri [50] showed that chronic pain negatively impacted the immune system. An immune response to chronic pain is the release of inflammatory substances such as antibodies, cytokines, and chemokines. When the immune system attacks the body, it results in inflammation of joints, which may cause pain, stiffness, and difficulties with mobility [51]. Inflammation contributes too many age-related degenerative joint diseases such as frailty, osteoporosis, atherosclerosis,

DOI: http://dx.doi.org/10.5772/intechopen.113974

type 2 diabetes, sarcopenia, and Alzheimer's disease [52]. Inflammation can be acute or chronic: acute inflammation will respond immediately to trauma due to injury, whereas chronic inflammation is slow, and long-term lasting [53].

With age, the risk of inflammation increases due to an unhealthy lifestyle, such as an unhealthy diet or physical inactivity. A review of studies conducted shows that, "...lifestyle interventions such as exercise training and dietary modifications may provide a low cost and long-term alternative to limit inflammation and slow declines in the elderly." [54].

According to Pahwa, et al., [53] 350 million people worldwide and almost 42 million Americans, suffer from arthritis and joint diseases of which osteoarthritis and osteoporosis occur more in menopausal women than older men [55]. As osteoarthritis is the most common age-related disorder in the world [56], the deterioration of the connective tissues that holds the joints together is found to be a major contributor to the development of osteoarthritis, which results in the increase of stiffness of ligaments and tendons [57]. To slow down the progression of osteoarthritis or osteoporosis, an exercise program that consists of spinal extensor strengthening with progressive measured resistance is recommended to prevent falls and fractures [58]. In addition to resistance training, movement to improve range of motion and overall functional performance should become a part of every aging adult. The Arthritis Foundation states the "movement is the best medicine for osteoarthritis."

Oxidative stress or reactive oxygen species (ROS) can cause chronic inflammation and affect a variety of physiological and pathological processes playing a role in age-related diseases like sarcopenia, cancer, cerebrovascular and neurodegenerative diseases. ROS induces cellular senescence eventually leading to cell death. Studies show that low to moderate levels of exercise-induced ROS production plays an essential role in exercise-induced adaptation of skeletal muscle [59]. Lack of exercise, suboptimal amount and quality of sleep, and poor diet all contribute to the accumulation of ROS. Homocysteine, an amino acid, influences ROS accumulation. There is evidence that elevated levels of homocysteine is associated with lower muscle strength in women and considered a risk factor for vascular and coronary heart disease. Recent studies report on the positive effects of Nordic walking (walking with poles mimicking the motion of cross- country skiing), reducing homocysteine levels and ensuring adequate supply of vitamin D. Vitamin D is essential for bone health and skeletal muscle function and continuously decreases over a lifetime. Vitamin D supplementation combined with outdoor activity in fresh air lowers homocysteine levels compared to supplementation alone.

There is growing evidence that depression is accompanied by increased levels of proinflammatory cytokines. This is based on a theory of a link between innate immunity and the central nervous system leading to decreased synthesis of serotonin and increased cortisol levels, characteristics of depressive conditions. Several studies have shown the benefits of movement and showed that regular physical activity improves immunity and may limit the effects or delay immunological aging. Regular aerobic exercise increases immune system function to prevent and defend against infection through reducing age-related increase in proinflammatory cytokines.

Recent genomic and functional studies suggest that immune and inflammation pathways are involved in the pathogenesis of Alzheimer's disease (AD) and Parkinson's disease (PD), the most common age-related neurodegenerative disorders. Both of these diseases are characterized by chronic inflammation in the brain. The chronic neuroinflammation compromises the blood–brain barrier (BBB) integrity, increasing its permeability and leading to loss of immunological protection of the central nervous system. There is body evidence that regular physical exercise has anti-inflammatory effects and reduces blood-brain barrier permeability reinforcing antioxidative capacity and reducing oxidative stress [60]. Furthermore, regular physical activity improves endothelial function and increases the density of brain capillaries. Therefore, physical training should be a component of prevention programs to reduce the risk of neuroinflammatory diseases.

Gentle stretching helps resolve inflammation and reduce pain. Stretching exercises and guided exercise programs with a prominent stretching component like Yoga, Tai-Chi and Essentrics have been found to decrease levels of circulating pro-inflammatory cytokines. Researchers from Harvard found that rats who were comfortably stretched for 10 minutes twice per day had better mobility (longer gait), less pain and reduced inflammatory infiltration in the connective tissues 2 weeks after pain injection. Furthermore, stretching also increased the rate of healing [30].

5. Movement and brain health

As we age, it is inevitable that not only our physical ability declines, but our cognitive ability declines, as well. As with physical impairment, cognitive impairment can be prevented and delayed. But what is cognition? Cognition is defined as "the mental action or process of acquiring knowledge and understanding through thought, experience, and the senses." [61]. Cognitive impairment in older adults can have many causes, including, but not limited to, the side effects of medication, infections, depression, dementia, and stress to name a few. A cohort study conducted by Kulsheshtha et al. [62] with 24,448 participants over the age of 45 found that there is an association between stress and cognitive impairment. Another study conducted in Sweden showed a significantly higher level of perceived stress in adults of advanced age [63]. Acute and chronic stress can result in oxidative stress, neuroinflammation and dysfunction of the blood–brain barrier leading to poor health outcomes. Anxiety and depression often accompany aging, increasing by up to 6% among those over the age of 65. Significant changes due to aging can cause feelings of insecurity, loss of self-esteem, anxiety and depression. Regular exercise therapy reduces stress and depression. In fact, studies show that running therapy was shown to have more beneficial effects on biological aging than antidepressant medications. Many studies have also shown the benefits of exercise in cognition. A literature review conducted by van Uffelen et al. [64] showed that exercising programs that included strength, flexibility, and balance training, improved cognition in both healthy older adults as well as older adults with cognitive decline. A study by Lautenschlager [65] reported that physical activity reduces the risk of cognitive decline later in life. Aspects of cognitive function that may be improved include memory, attention, executive function (the ability to plan and organize; monitor, inhibit, or facilitate behaviors; initiate tasks; and control emotions).

The protection of the aging brain and the central nervous system from neurodegeneration poses significant challenges. In addition to apparent physical changes due to aging, there are often equally significant changes in the brain and in mental health. The brain shrinks in volume, particularly in the frontal cortex and its weight declines with age at a rate of around 5% per decade after age 40. The white matter found in the deeper tissues of the brain that contain nerve fibers wrapped by a fatty sheath called myelin deteriorates after around the age of 40. Memory loss is the most widely seen cognitive change associated with aging. There are four sections that comprise memory functioning: episodic, semantic, procedural and working memory. Loss of episodic memory characterizes memory loss in Alzheimer's disease. Several studies demonstrated that physical activity, especially aerobic exercise performed by elderly people is protective against Alzheimer's disease, slowing the decline in cognition and slows disease progression through reducing amyloid-B level deposition. On the other hand, sedentary life patterns and lack of physical activity increase the risk of dementia and Alzheimer's disease [66].

There is a growing interest in the gut-brain axis and there is accumulating evidence that the gut microbiota is critical to health and disease. Dysbiosis, a term for poor gut health, is characterized by microbiota dysregulation and results in an unbalanced microbiome in the gut. A healthy microbiome (symbiosis) promotes overall health. The gut-brain axis is the bidirectional link between the central nervous system (CNS) and the enteric nervous system (ENS). It seems like an "unhealthy gut" can lead to an "unhealthy brain". Dysbiosis is associated with neurodegenerative diseases including Alzheimer's, Parkinson's, Huntington's, and multiple sclerosis. For example, a review conducted by Ref. [67, 68] highlighted the role of Vitamin D deficiency or hypovitaminosis D among patients with Parkinson's disease due to a deterioration in the gastrointestinal function. Furthermore, the paper also states that neurodegenerative diseases and hypovitaminosis D led to frailty, a concept that has grown in importance in understanding the functional status of older adults' health. Frailty is a condition of risk and vulnerability diminished resistance to stressors and is associated with poor gut health [68]. Meanwhile, there is compelling evidence that shows many different types of exercise not only enhance cognitive functioning but provide a promising role for neurodegenerative diseases [1]. Exercise has been shown to increase the diversity of the microbiota, balancing beneficial and pathogenic bacterial communities and enhance colon health. Regular physical activity also increases butyrate-producing bacteria critical for maintaining the mucosal barrier, modulating immune response, preventing infections and regulating energy expenditure. Furthermore, exercise increases both endogenous and exogenous production of vitamin D which further increases the capacity to exercise.

Brain-derived neurotrophic factor (BDNF), a key protein molecule involved in learning and memory, decreases with aging. BDNF is also considered as the main player in brain plasticity. Movement, particularly aerobic and resistance exercise and endurance activity plays a neuroprotective role by increasing BDNF production [68]. Some studies indicate that exercise improves neuropsychiatric and cognitive symptoms in people with mental disorders. Interestingly, these studies show that the delivery of exogenous BDNF into the patient's brain had no therapeutic effect on the disease but releasing BDNF through physical activity was neuroprotective. Irisin, commonly referred to as the "sport hormone" is released from muscle cells after physical activity that induces oxygen consumption and heat production. Irisin protects against neuroinflammation by acting directly on glial cells in the brain, reducing oxidative and physiological stress, and protects against cerebral ischemia [1].

Regular physical activity provides a variety of other benefits, including helping people sleep better, feel better, and perform daily tasks more easily. There is a bidirectional relationship between sleep and exercise. Studies demonstrate that moderate to vigorous physical activity improves quality of sleep among adults. On the other hand, insufficient or poor quality of sleep leads to lower levels of physical activity. Regular physical activity reduces the length of time it takes to go to sleep, reduces the time one is awake after going to sleep and before rising in the morning and lengthens deep sleep. Exercise is also used to treat sleeping disorders. For example, 4 months of aerobic exercise training in a sample of older adults with insomnia significantly improved sleep quality while also reducing daytime sleepiness and depressive symptoms. Another research study found that 12 weeks of moderate-intensity aerobic and resistance exercise resulted in a 25% reduction in obstructive sleep apnea (OSA) severity despite less than 1 kg of weight loss [69]. Indeed, regular exercise leads to better subjective and objective sleep and improvements in daytime functioning.

6. Recommendations

Past studies have aimed to determine an ideal movement program for older adults to combat changes in aging. Combining scientific support and motivational attributes, educating adults about the type and dose of movement in quality of life both before and at the onset of such reductions is critical [6]. Various forms of movement have all shown to be beneficial in some way in countering various weaknesses from aging, whether it be resistance training [70], endurance training and concurrent strength [71], Tai Chi [72, 73], multidimensional exercise training [7], functional training [74], dance [75], vibration therapy [76, 77], dynamic stretching [78–80] and static stretching [78, 81].

Both medical professionals and community/public health programs are essential in promoting movement as prevention and treatment. This ideology is the foundation for the American College of Sport Medicine (ACSM) Exercise is Medicine global initiative. ACSM and Health Level Seven International (HL7), a global health care database network approved a Physical Activity Implementation Guide that includes physical activity as a vital sign to facilitate health care professionals providing referrals to exercise professionals [82]. The Physical Activity Guidelines for Americans (2018) recommends that adults should move more and sit less throughout the day acknowledging that some physical activity is better than none. Furthermore, it recommends that at least 150 minutes (2.5 hours) to 300 minutes (5 hours) a week of moderate intensity or 75 minutes (1 hour and 15 minutes) to 150 minutes (2 hours and 30 minutes) a week of vigorous-intensity aerobic physical activity, or an equivalent combination of moderate- and vigorous-intensity aerobic activity will lead to substantial benefits and even more additional health benefits beyond 300 minutes (5 hours). Recommendations for older adults (aged 65 and older) are the same but with additional elements of including multicomponent physical activity that emphasizes balance training, aerobics, and muscle-strengthening activities at moderate or greater intensity on 3 or more days a week to enhance functional capacity and to prevent falls. These recommendations align with the WHO recommendations (**Table 1**, **Figures 1–3**).

The intensity of exercise is based on absolute rates of energy expenditure commonly described as light, moderate, or vigorous intensity. Light intensity activity is non-sedentary waking behavior including walking at a slow or leisurely pace (2 mph or less), cooking activities, or light household chores. Moderate intensity activity includes activities like walking briskly (2.5 to 4 mph), playing doubles tennis, or raking the yard. Vigorous intensity activity samples include jogging, running, carrying heavy groceries or other loads upstairs, shoveling snow, or participating in a strenuous fitness class.

Aerobic physical activity is also classified into levels: inactive, insufficiently active, active, and highly active. The classifications are useful to help one determine his/her level and how to work on becoming more active. Inactive is basic movement derived

- Older adults should do at least 150–300 minutes of moderate-intensity aerobic physical activity; or at least 75–150 minutes of vigorous-intensity aerobic physical activity; or an equivalent combination of moderate- and vigorous-intensity activity throughout the week, for substantial health benefits.
- Older adults should also do muscle-strengthening activities at moderate or greater intensity that involve all major muscle groups on 2 or more days a week, as these provide additional health benefits.
- As part of their weekly physical activity, older adults should do varied multicomponent physical activity that emphasizes functional balance and strength training at moderate or greater intensity, on 3 or more days a week, to enhance functional capacity and to prevent falls.

Table 1.
WHO guidelines for physical activity and sedentary behavior for older adults.

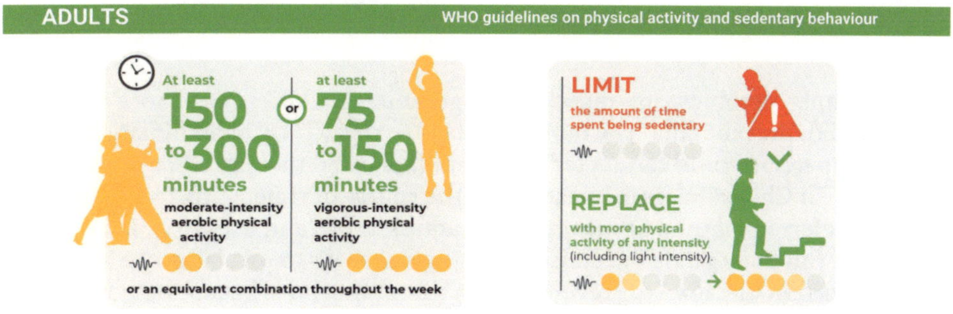

Figure 1.
WHO guidelines on physical activity and sedentary behavior for adults.

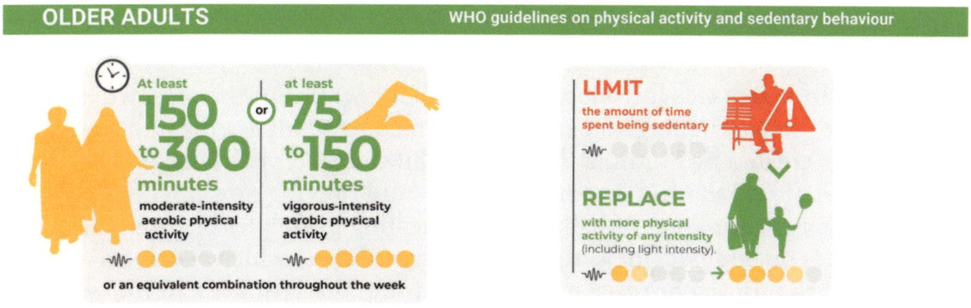

Figure 2.
WHO guidelines on physical activity and sedentary behavior for older adults.

from daily life activities. Insufficiently active is doing some moderate- or vigorous-intensity physical activity but less than 150 minutes of moderate-intensity physical activity a week or 75 minutes of vigorous-intensity physical activity or the equivalent combination. This level is less than the target range for meeting the key guidelines for adults. Active is doing the equivalent of 150 minutes to 300 minutes of moderate-intensity physical activity a week. This level meets the key guideline target range for adults. Highly active is doing the equivalent of more than 300 minutes of moderate-intensity physical activity a week. This level exceeds the key guideline target range for adults.

Guided exercise programs provide opportunities for older adults to meet the additional elements of including multicomponent physical activity that emphasizes

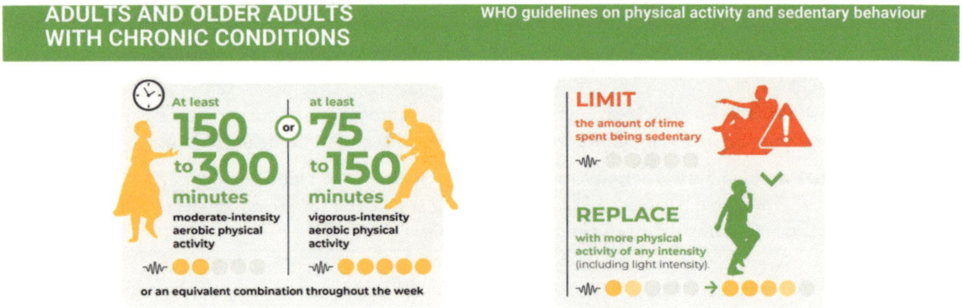

Figure 3.
WHO guidelines on physical activity and sedentary behavior for adults with chronic conditions.

balance training, aerobics, and muscle-strengthening activities to enhance functional capacity and to prevent falls. The most popular are Yoga, Tai-Chi and Pilates. A 10-year comparison study conducted in Australia showed that participation in Yoga, Pilates, and Tai Chi exercises increased over the course of time, with Yoga and Pilates being the preferred method of movement in adults age 55 and over [83]. Recently, Essentrics, a full body guided exercise program that seeks to rebalance the body was introduced in Canada as a "reverse aging" program and is becoming popular. Essentrics may have the most potential benefits and the least number of side effects because of its gentle approach and focus on aging. Although there are differences between these guided exercise programs all forms of movement are designed to improve physical and mental health using a full body approach.

6.1 Essentrics

A holistic approach was introduced as a full body work-out that uses a dynamic combination of strengthening and stretching aimed to rebalance the body. Essentrics was created by Miranda Esmonde-White a former ballerina with the National Ballet of Canada and draws on the slow and flowing movements of Tai-Chi, the strengthening techniques of ballet and the healing principles of physiotherapy. Essentrics relies on bodyweight as the source of resistance, which contrasts with traditional strength training or resistance training programs that use external weights. The movement sequences of Essentrics consist of low impact full body stretches emphasizing alignment to loosen and decompress the joints and relax the muscles. A study conducted by Zarco et al. [79] included older adults who participated in a guided exercise program, which showed an improved flexibility, balance, and strength (**Figures 4** and 5).

6.2 Yoga

The practice of yoga was developed in Northern India around 2700 BC and offers physical benefits as well as mental wellness [84]. It is a type of exercise in which the body moves into various positions to become more fit or flexible, to improve breathing, and relax the mind. There are many different types of yoga in the world, but "Hatha Yoga" is the most popular in the West [85]. Blending western gymnastic styles with classic yoga became very popular. Since, the United Nations Assembly

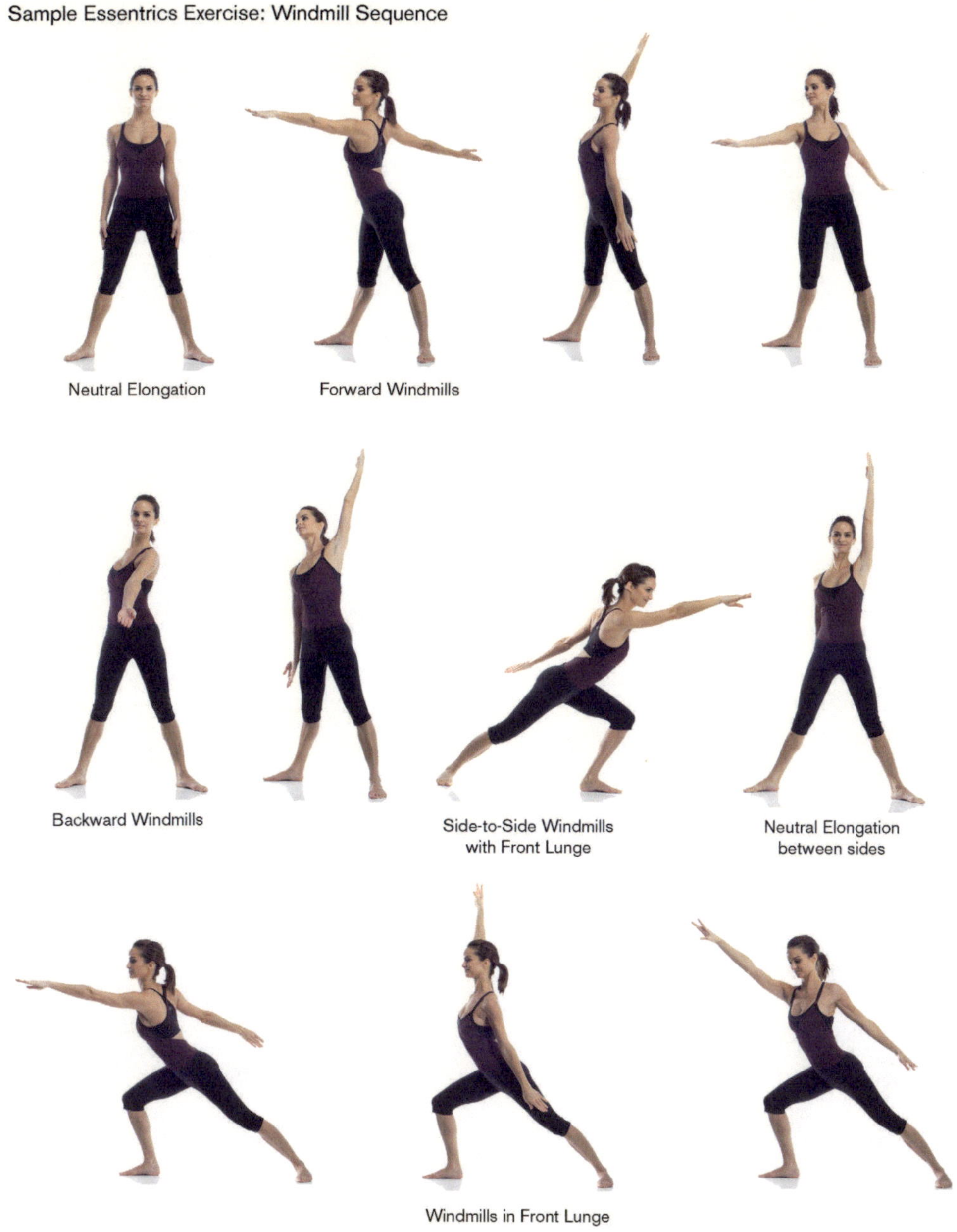

Figure 4.
Essentrics sample exercise - windmill sequence.

announced an "International Day of Yoga," in 2015, and UNESCO claimed yoga as an "intangible cultural heritage" [84]. The benefits of yoga include increased joint flexibility and joint function, and with regular practice it can reduce joint pain [86]. In a randomized control study conducted by [87] yoga improved flexibility, strength, and balance in older adults. Yoga is especially recommended for aging-related chronic ailments [88].

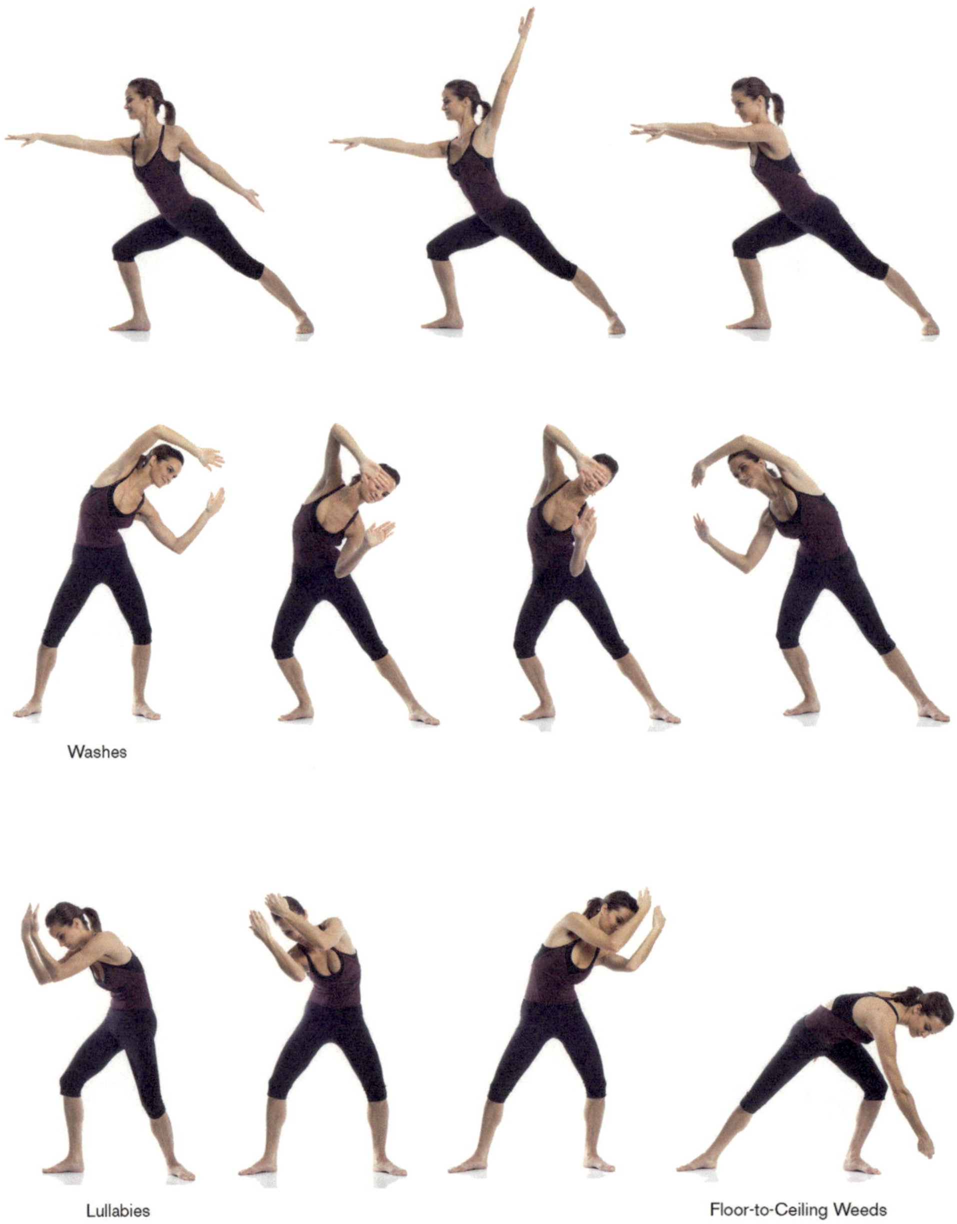

Figure 5.
Sample Essentrics exercise - washes and lullabies sequence.

6.3 Tai Chi

Another form of complementary therapy is Tai Chi. Tai Chi is a form of Chinese martial arts. It was developed around 1670 by Chen Wangting as a method for self-defense but has shown to have great health benefits [89]. Tai Chi is a type of exercise where different postures and flowing movements result in attaining optimal physiological and psychological benefits [90]. Tai Chi is used to manage chronic pain conditions since slow motion and weight shifting may improve musculoskeletal strength and joint stability. A review of studies showed that a 24-week Tai Chi exercise program for patients diagnosed with osteoporosis resulted in reduced pain, particularly in reduced lower back pain [91].

6.4 Pilates

Joseph H. Pilates developed these exercises in the 1920s as a method of conditioning ballet and modern dancers. Pilates is defined as an exercise regimen that is typically performed on a floor mat or with the use of a specialized apparatus and aims to improve flexibility and stability by strengthening the muscles, especially torso-stabilizing muscles of the abdomen and lower back. It focuses on controlled movement, posture, and breathing [92] A review conducted by [93] showed that the Pilates method reduces the risk of falls in older adults and improves balance and mobility.

These guided exercise programs share the same fundamental goal of mastering control over lifting and moving the body in space, are low impact and use the body weight as the resistance force for strengthening. Furthermore, they all utilize synchronized breathing with movements and varying degrees of body and mindful awareness. Studies on Pilates, Yoga, and Tai Chi have all had significant effects on the improvement of strength, body composition and flexibility. Furthermore, studies on Yoga and Pilates show it's beneficial in reducing inflammation. Pilates strengthens the bones and joints while yoga helps to build and increase the flexibility of the muscles around the joints [94]. Studies on Tai Chi show that it improves balance because of increased joint stability and postural control. There are few studies on Essentrics but initial studies show improvements in balance, strength, flexibility and address pain (**Table 2**).

It has been generally accepted that a reduction in functional capabilities is just a natural part of aging. However, more recent ideologies suggest that changes in functionality are not simply due to mere aging but increasing sedentariness or an inactive lifestyle. Distinguishing inevitable age-related changes versus those resulting

Be active		**Sit less**	**Build strength**	**Improve balance**
Vigorous	**Moderate**		**Improve functional mobility**	
Run Play Sports Climb Stairs	Walk Cycle Swim	Limit Sitting Time, Sofa Time and Computer Time	Weight Training Essentrics Yoga Pilates	Dance Tai Chi Essentrics Bowls
A total of 75 minutes of vigorous intensity or 150 minutes of moderate intensity or a combination of both PER WEEK		Break up sitting time per day	2 days or more PER WEEK	
10-30 or more minutes per session per day			10-30 minutes or more per session per day	
		Something is better than nothing.		
		Start small and build up gradually.		

Table 2.
Suggested physical activities or guided exercise programs for aging adults.

from inactivity are critical for preserving quality of life. It is inevitable that aging and slowing down go hand and hand. However, this linkage is largely a result of a sedentary lifestyle. There is overwhelming evidence that the body is capable of responding to exercise throughout one's life and gives hope to all that effective movement may be sustained as we age. Although it's never too late, learning movement skills early in life will assist in maintenance with greater ease over the life span. Undeniably, movement, physical activity and exercise benefit aging and streamlining technology-based analyses, conducting research at the cellular and molecular levels and pinpointing interventions is the wave of future directions.

Author details

Emilia Patricia Zarco*, Anne Gibbone and Hanna Matatyaho
Adelphi University, Garden City, NY, USA

*Address all correspondence to: zarco@adelphi.edu

References

[1] Bičíková M, Máčová L, Jandová D, Třískala Z, Hill M. Movement as a positive modulator of aging. International Journal of Molecular Sciences [Internet]. 2021;**22**(12):6278. Available from: https://www.ncbi.nlm.nih.gov/pmc/articles/PMC8230594

[2] World Health Organisation. The Global Status Report on Physical Activity 2022 [Internet]. www.who.int. 2022. Available from: https://www.who.int/teams/health-promotion/physical-activity/global-status-report-on-physical-activity-2022

[3] CDC. Why Should People be Active? [Internet]. Centers for Disease Control and Prevention. 2020. Available from: https://www.cdc.gov/physicalactivity/activepeoplehealthynation/why-should-people-be-active.html

[4] LaMonte MJ, Lewis CE, Buchner DM, Evenson KR, Rillamas-Sun E, Di C, et al. Both light intensity and moderate-to-vigorous physical activity measured by Accelerometry are Favorably associated with Cardiometabolic risk factors in older women: The objective physical activity and cardiovascular health (OPACH) study. Journal of the American Heart Association. 2017;**6**(10)

[5] Woodcock J, Franco OH, Orsini N, Roberts I. Non-vigorous physical activity and all-cause mortality: Systematic review and meta-analysis of cohort studies. International Journal of Epidemiology [Internet]. 2010;**40**(1):121-138. Available from: https://academic.oup.com/ije/article/40/1/121/658816

[6] Szychowska A, Drygas W. Physical activity as a determinant of successful aging: A narrative review article. Aging Clinical and Experimental Research. 2021;**34**(6):1209-1214

[7] Pepera G, Krinta K, Mpea C, Antoniou V, Peristeropoulos A, Dimitriadis Z. Randomized controlled trial of group exercise intervention for fall risk factors reduction in nursing home residents. Canadian Journal on Aging / La Revue canadienne du vieillissement. 2022;**11**:1-9

[8] Volpi E, Nazemi R, Fujita S. Muscle tissue changes with aging. Current opinion in clinical nutrition and metabolic care [Internet]. 2004;**7**(4):405-410. Available from: https://www.ncbi.nlm.nih.gov/pmc/articles/PMC2804956/

[9] Locquet M, Beaudart C, Bruyère O, Kanis JA, Delandsheere L, Reginster JY. Bone health assessment in older people with or without muscle health impairment. Osteoporosis International. 2018;**29**(5):1057-1067

[10] Ramsey KA, Rojer AGM, D'Andrea L, Otten RHJ, Heymans MW, Trappenburg MC, et al. The association of objectively measured physical activity and sedentary behavior with skeletal muscle strength and muscle power in older adults: A systematic review and meta-analysis. Ageing Research Reviews. 2021;**67**:101266

[11] Lu L, Mao L, Feng Y, Ainsworth BE, Liu Y, Chen N. Effects of different exercise training modes on muscle strength and physical performance in older people with sarcopenia: A systematic review and meta-analysis. BMC Geriatrics. 2021;**21**(1)

[12] Zoico E, Di Francesco V, Guralnik JM, Mazzali G, Bortolani A, Guariento S, et al. Physical disability

and muscular strength in relation to obesity and different body composition indexes in a sample of healthy elderly women. International Journal of Obesity and Related Metabolic Disorders: Journal of the International Association for the Study of Obesity [Internet]. 2004;**28**(2):234-241. Available from: https://pubmed.ncbi.nlm.nih.gov/14708033/

[13] Nantel J, Mathieu ME, Prince F. Physical activity and obesity: Biomechanical and physiological key concepts. Journal of Obesity [Internet]. 2011;**2011**:1-10. Available from: https://www.ncbi.nlm.nih.gov/pmc/articles/PMC2990021/

[14] Forhan M, Gill SV. Obesity, functional mobility and quality of life. Best Practice & Research Clinical Endocrinology & Metabolism. 2013;**27**:129-137. Available from: https://scirp.org/reference/ReferencesPapers.aspx?ReferenceID=1924535

[15] Sharma L, Hurwitz DE, Thonar EJ-MA, Sum JA, Lenz ME, Dunlop DD, et al. Knee adduction moment, serum hyaluronan level, and disease severity in medial tibiofemoral osteoarthritis. Arthritis and Rheumatism. 1998;**41**(7):1233-1240

[16] Wearing SC, Hennig EM, Byrne NM, Steele JR, Hills AP. Musculoskeletal disorders associated with obesity: A biomechanical perspective. Obesity Reviews [Internet]. 2006;7(3):239-250. Available from: https://onlinelibrary.wiley.com/doi/abs/10.1111/j.1467-789X.2006.00251.x

[17] Bergen G, Stevens MR, Burns ER. Falls and fall injuries among adults aged ≥65 years — United States, 2014. MMWR Morbidity and Mortality Weekly Report. 2016;**65**(37):993-998

[18] Zanotto T, Chen L, Fang J, Bhattacharya SB, Alexander NB, Sosnoff JJ. Minimizing fall-related injuries in at-risk older adults: The falling safely training (FAST) study protocol. Contemporary Clinical Trials Communications [Internet]. 2023;**33**:101133. Available from: https://www.sciencedirect.com/science/article/pii/S2451865423000790

[19] Dautzenberg L, Beglinger S, Tsokani S, Zevgiti S, Raijmann RCMA, Rodondi N, et al. Interventions for preventing falls and fall-related fractures in community-dwelling older adults: A systematic review and network meta-analysis. Journal of the American Geriatrics Society. 2021;**69**(10):2973-2984

[20] Sherrington C, Fairhall N, Wallbank G, Tiedemann A, Michaleff ZA, Howard K, et al. Exercise for preventing falls in older people living in the community: An abridged Cochrane systematic review. British Journal of Sports Medicine. Aug 2020;**54**(15):885-891. DOI: 10.1136/bjsports-2019-101512. Epub 2019 Dec 2. PMID: 31792067

[21] Thomas E, Battaglia G, Patti A, Brusa J, Leonardi V, Palma A, et al. Physical activity programs for balance and fall prevention in elderly. Medicine [Internet]. 2019;**98**(27):e16218. Available from: https://www.ncbi.nlm.nih.gov/pmc/articles/PMC6635278/

[22] Lord SR, Clark RD. Simple physiological and clinical tests for the accurate prediction of falling in older people. Gerontology. 1996;**42**(4):199-203

[23] Cruz-Jimenez M. Normal changes in gait and mobility problems in the elderly. Physical Medicine and Rehabilitation Clinics of North America. 2017;**28**(4):713-725

[24] Cebolla EC, Rodacki ALF, Bento PCB. Balance, gait, functionality and strength: Comparison between elderly fallers and non-fallers. Brazilian Journal of Physical Therapy [Internet]. 2015;**19**(2):146-151. Available from: https://www.ncbi.nlm.nih.gov/pmc/articles/PMC4481835/

[25] Kyrdalen IL, Thingstad P, Sandvik L, Ormstad H. Associations between gait speed and well-known fall risk factors among community-dwelling older adults. Physiotherapy Research International. 2018;**24**(1):e1743

[26] Kwon MS, Kwon YR, Park YS, Kim JW. Comparison of gait patterns in elderly fallers and non-fallers. Gómez C, Schwarzacher SP, Zhou H, editors. Technology and Health Care. 2018;**26**:427-436

[27] Behm DG, Cavanaugh T, Quigley P, Reid JC, Nardi PSM, Marchetti PH. Acute bouts of upper and lower body static and dynamic stretching increase non-local joint range of motion. European Journal of Applied Physiology. 2015;**116**(1):241-249

[28] Chaouachi A, Padulo J, Kasmi S, Othmen AB, Chatra M, Behm DG. Unilateral static and dynamic hamstrings stretching increases contralateral hip flexion range of motion. Clinical Physiology and Functional Imaging. 2015;**37**(1):23-29

[29] Wilke J, Macchi V, De Caro R, Stecco C. Fascia thickness, aging and flexibility: Is there an association? Journal of Anatomy. 2018;**234**(1):43-49

[30] Langevin HM. Connective tissue: A body-wide signaling network? Medical Hypotheses. 2006;**66**(6):1074-1077

[31] Collier R. A short history of pain management. Canadian Medical Association Journal. 2018;**190**(1):E26-E27

[32] American Society of Anesthesiologists. What are opioids?—Made for this moment [internet]. Made for this moment | Anesthesia. Pain Management & Surgery. 2021. Available from: https://www.asahq.org/madeforthismoment/pain-management/opioid-treatment/what-are-opioids/

[33] Raja SN, Carr DB, Cohen M, Finnerup NB, Flor H, Gibson S, et al. The revised International Association for the Study of Pain definition of pain: Concepts, challenges, and compromises. Pain. 2020;**5**:1976-1982. Articles in Press(9)

[34] Geneen LJ, Moore RA, Clarke C, Martin D, Colvin LA, Smith BH. Physical activity and exercise for chronic pain in adults: An overview of Cochrane reviews. Cochrane Database of Systematic Reviews [Internet]. 2017;**4**(4) Available from: https://www.ncbi.nlm.nih.gov/pmc/articles/PMC5461882/

[35] Patel KV, Guralnik JM, Dansie EJ, Turk DC. Prevalence and impact of pain among older adults in the United States: Findings from the 2011 National Health and aging trends study. Pain. 2013;**154**(12):2649-2657

[36] Hosseini F, Mullins S, Gibson W, Thake M. Acute pain management for older adults. Clinical Medicine. 2022;**22**(4):302-306

[37] Goldberg DS, McGee SJ. Pain as a global public health priority. BMC Public Health [Internet]. 2011;**11**(1) Available from: https://bmcpublichealth.biomedcentral.com/articles/10.1186/1471-2458-11-770

[38] GSK Consumer Healthcare Global Pain Index Report 4 th edition -2020 [Internet]. Available from: https://www.gsk.com/media/6351/2020-global-plain-index-report.pdf

[39] Rikard SM. Chronic pain among adults—United States, 2019-2021. MMWR Morbidity and Mortality Weekly Report [Internet]. 2023;**72**:379-385. Available from: https://www.cdc.gov/mmwr/volumes/72/wr/mm7215a1.htm

[40] Chronic pain prevalence among adults by age U.S. 2019 [Internet]. Statista. Available from: https://www.statista.com/statistics/1189525/chronic-pain-adults-prevalence-by-age-us/

[41] Vos T, Allen C, Arora M, Barber RM, Bhutta ZA, Brown A, et al. Global, regional, and national incidence, prevalence, and years lived with disability for 310 diseases and injuries, 1990-2015: A systematic analysis for the global burden of disease study 2015. The Lancet [Internet]. 2016;**388**(10053):1545-1602. Available from: https://www.ncbi.nlm.nih.gov/pmc/articles/PMC5055577/

[42] Han C, Pae CU. Pain and depression: A neurobiological perspective of their relationship. Psychiatry Investigation. 2015;**12**(1):1

[43] Merkle SL, Sluka KA, Frey-Law LA. The interaction between pain and movement. Journal of Hand Therapy. 2020;**33**(1):60-66

[44] Hodges PW, Smeets RJ. Interaction between pain, movement, and physical activity. The Clinical Journal of Pain. 2015;**31**(2):97-107

[45] Mior S. Exercise in the treatment of chronic pain. The Clinical Journal of Pain. 2001;**17**(Supplement):S77-S85

[46] Heneweer H, Vanhees L, Picavet SJH. Physical activity and low back pain: A U-shaped relation? Pain [Internet]. 2009;**143**(1):21-25. Available from: https://www.sciencedirect.com/science/article/pii/S0304395908007719

[47] Landmark T, Romundstad PR, Borchgrevink PC, Kaasa S, Dale O. Longitudinal associations between exercise and pain in the general population - the HUNT pain study. PLoS One. 2013;**8**(6):e65279

[48] Weyand CM, Goronzy JJ. Aging of the immune system. Mechanisms and therapeutic targets. Annals of the American Thoracic Society [Internet]. 2016;**13**(Supplement_5):S422-S428. Available from: https://www.ncbi.nlm.nih.gov/pmc/articles/PMC5291468/

[49] Marshall JS, Warrington R, Watson W, Kim HL. An introduction to immunology and immunopathology. Allergy, Asthma & Clinical Immunology [Internet]. 2018;**14**(S2) Available from: https://aacijournal.biomedcentral.com/articles/10.1186/s13223-018-0278

[50] Does Chronic Pain Really Weaken our Immune System? - SAPNA Pain Management Blog [Internet]. Spine and Pain Clinics of North America. 2020. Available from: https://www.sapnamed.com/blog/does-chronic-pain-really-weaken-our-immune-system/

[51] Orlowsky EW, Kraus VB. The role of innate immunity in osteoarthritis: When our first line of Defense goes on the offensive. The Journal of Rheumatology [Internet]. 2015;**42**(3):363-371. Available from: https://www.ncbi.nlm.nih.gov/pmc/articles/PMC4465583/

[52] Rezuș E, Cardoneanu A, Burlui A, Luca A, Codreanu C, Tamba BI, et al. The link between Inflammaging and

degenerative joint diseases. International Journal of Molecular Sciences [Internet]. 2019;**20**(3):614. Available from: https://www.mdpi.com/1422-0067/20/3/614

[53] Pahwa R, Jialal I. Chronic Inflammation [Internet]. NIH.gov. StatPearls Publishing; 2019. Available from: https://www.ncbi.nlm.nih.gov/books/NBK493173/

[54] Woods JA, Wilund KR, Martin SA, Kistler BM. Exercise, inflammation and aging. Aging and disease [Internet]. 2012;**3**(1):130-140. Available from: https://www.ncbi.nlm.nih.gov/pmc/articles/PMC3320801/

[55] Ji MX, Yu Q. Primary osteoporosis in postmenopausal women. Chronic Diseases and Translational Medicine [Internet]. 2015;**1**(1):9-13. Available from: https://www.ncbi.nlm.nih.gov/pmc/articles/PMC5643776/

[56] Shane Anderson A, Loeser RF. Why is osteoarthritis an age-related disease? Best Practice & Research Clinical Rheumatology. 2010;**24**(1):15-26

[57] Tu M, Yao Y, Qiao F, Wang L. The pathogenic role of connective tissue growth factor in osteoarthritis. Bioscience Reports [Internet]. 2019;**39**(7) Available from: https://portlandpress.com/bioscirep/article/39/7/BSR20191374/219330/The-pathogenic-role-of-connective-tissue-growth

[58] Sinaki M. Exercise for patients with osteoporosis: Management of Vertebral Compression Fractures and Trunk Strengthening for fall prevention. PM&R. 2012;**4**(11):882-888

[59] Exercise-induced oxidative stress. Friend or foe? Journal of Sport and Health Science [Internet]. 2020;**9**(5):415-425. Available from: https://www.sciencedirect.com/science/article/pii/S2095254620300

[60] Małkiewicz MA, Szarmach A, Sabisz A, Cubała WJ, Szurowska E, Winklewski PJ. Blood-brain barrier permeability and physical exercise. Journal of Neuroinflammation. 2019;**16**(1)

[61] Mak Y. What is cognition? [Internet] Cambridge Cognition. 2015. Available from: https://cambridgecognition.com/what-is-cognition/#:~:text=Cognition%20is%20defined%20as%20

[62] Kulshreshtha A, Alonso A, McClure LA, Hajjar I, Manly JJ, Judd S. Association of Stress with Cognitive Function among Older Black and White US adults. JAMA Network Open [Internet]. 2023;**6**(3):e231860. Available from: https://jamanetwork.com/journals/jamanetworkopen/fullarticle/2802090?utm_campaign=articlePDF&utm_medium=articlePDFlink&utm_source=articlePDF&utm_content=jamanetworkopen.2023.1860

[63] Osmanovic-Thunström A, Mossello E, Åkerstedt T, Fratiglioni L, Wang HX. Do levels of perceived stress increase with increasing age after age 65? A population-based study. Age and Ageing [Internet]. 2015;**44**(5):828-834. Available from: https://academic.oup.com/ageing/article/44/5/828/52059

[64] Van Uffelen M, Mechelen V. The effects of exercise on cognition in older adults with and without cognitive decline: A systematic review. Clinical Journal of Sport Medicine. 2008;**18**: 486-500. [Internet]. Available from: https://vuir.vu.edu.au/24174/1/van%20Uffelen_Clin%20J%20Sports%20Med_PA%20and%20cognition%20systematic%20review.pdf

[65] Lautenschlager NT, Almeida OP. Physical activity and cognition in old age. Current Opinion in Psychiatry. 2006;**19**(2):190-193

[66] Yan S, Fu W, Wang C, Mao J, Liu B, Zou L, et al. Association between sedentary behavior and the risk of dementia: A systematic review and meta-analysis. Translational Psychiatry. 2020;**10**(1)

[67] Sleiman SF, Henry J, Al-Haddad R, El Hayek L, Abou Haidar E, Stringer T, et al. Exercise promotes the expression of brain derived neurotrophic factor (BDNF) through the action of the ketone body β-hydroxybutyrate. eLife [Internet]. 2016;**5**:e15092. Available from: https://www.ncbi.nlm.nih.gov/pmc/articles/PMC4915811/

[68] Palermo S, Stanziano M, Nigri A, Civilotti C, Celeghin A. Parkinson's disease, SARS-CoV-2, and frailty: Is there a vicious cycle related to Hypovitaminosis D? Brain Sciences [Internet]. 2023;**13**(4):528. Available from: https://pubmed.ncbi.nlm.nih.gov/37190492/

[69] Kline CE. The bidirectional relationship between exercise and sleep. American Journal of Lifestyle Medicine. 2014;**8**(6):375-379

[70] Islam MR, Valaris S, Young MF, Haley EB, Luo R, Bond SF, et al. Exercise hormone irisin is a critical regulator of cognitive function. Nature Metabolism. 2021;**3**(8):1058-1070

[71] Valenzuela T. Efficacy of progressive resistance training interventions in older adults in nursing homes: A systematic review. Journal of the American Medical Directors Association. 2012;**13**(5):418-428

[72] Markov A, Hauser L, Chaabene H. Effects of concurrent strength and endurance training on measures of physical fitness in healthy middle-aged and older adults: A systematic review with meta-analysis. Sports Medicine. 2023;**53**(2):437-455

[73] Huang CY, Mayer PK, Wu MY, Liu DH, Wu PC, Yen HR. The effect of tai chi in elderly individuals with sarcopenia and frailty: A systematic review and meta-analysis of randomized controlled trials. Ageing Research Reviews. 2022;**82**:101747

[74] Wang X, Hu J, Wu D. Risk factors for frailty in older adults. Medicine [Internet]. 2022;**101**(34):e30169. Available from: https://www.ncbi.nlm.nih.gov/pmc/articles/PMC9410572/

[75] Bray NW, Smart RR, Jakobi JM, Jones GR. Exercise prescription to reverse frailty. Applied Physiology, Nutrition, and Metabolism. 2016;**41**(10):1112-1116

[76] Cox L, Youmans-Jones J. Dance is a healing art. Current Treatment Options in Allergy. 2023;**4**:1-12

[77] Tan J, Shi X, Witchalls J, Waddington G, Lun Fu AC, Wu S, et al. Effects of pre-exercise acute vibration training on symptoms of exercise-induced muscle damage. Journal of Strength and Conditioning Research. 2020;**36**(8):2339-2348

[78] Wu S, Ning HT, Xiao SM, Hu MY, Wu XY, Deng HW, et al. Effects of vibration therapy on muscle mass, muscle strength and physical function in older adults with sarcopenia: A systematic review and meta-analysis. European Review of Aging and Physical Activity. 2020;**17**(1)

[79] Chapman-Lopez TJ, Moris JM, Petty G, Timon C, Koh Y. Effects of static contemporary Western yoga vs. a dynamic stretching exercise program

on body composition. Balance, and Flexibility. 2022;**37**(5):1064-1069

[80] Zarco EPT, Aquino M, Petrizzo J, Wygand J, McGorry A. Perceived benefits of a guided exercise program among older adults. Gerontology and Geriatric Medicine. 2021;7:233372142110601

[81] Zarco EP, Aquino M, Petrizzo J, Wygand J, King JL. The impact of a 10-week Essentrics program on strength. Flexibility and Body Composition. 2022;**28**(2):75-84

[82] Arntz F, Markov A, Behm DG, Behrens M, Negra Y, Nakamura M, et al. Chronic effects of static stretching exercises on muscle strength and power in healthy individuals across the lifespan: A systematic review with multi-level meta-analysis. Sports Medicine. 2023;**53**(3):723-745

[83] News Detail [Internet]. ACSM_CMS. 2023. Available from: https://www.acsm.org/news-detail/2023/05/05/acsm-eim-achieve-major-victory-for-exercise-professionals-health-care

[84] Vergeer I, Bennie JA, Charity MJ, Harvey JT, van Uffelen JGZ, Biddle SJH, et al. Participation trends in holistic movement practices: A 10-year comparison of yoga/Pilates and t'ai chi/qigong use among a national sample of 195,926 Australians. BMC Complementary and Alternative Medicine. 2017;**17**(1)

[85] published RAD. When did yoga originate? [Internet]. livescience.com. 2021. Available from: https://www.livescience.com/when-did-yoga-originate

[86] Garfinkel M, Schumacher HR. YOGA. Rheumatic Disease Clinics of North America [Internet]. 2000;**26**(1):125-132. Available from: https://www.sciencedirect.com/science/article/pii/S0889857X05701265

[87] Yoga Benefits for Arthritis [Internet]. Available from: https://www.arthritis.org/health-wellness/healthy-living/physical-activity/yoga/yoga-benefits-for-arthritis

[88] Bucht D. Sauna yoga superiorly improves flexibility, strength, and balance: A two-armed randomized controlled trial in healthy older adults. International Journal of Environmental Research and Public Health. 2019;**16**(19):3721

[89] Gothe NP, McAuley E. Yoga is as good as stretching–strengthening exercises in improving functional fitness outcomes: Results from a randomized controlled trial. The Journals of Gerontology Series A: Biological Sciences and Medical Sciences [Internet]. 2015;**71**(3):406-411. Available from: https://academic.oup.com/biomedgerontology/article/71/3/406/2605263

[90] Lam P. History of Tai Chi | Tai Chi for Health Institute [internet]. Tai Chi for Health Institute. 2018. Available from: https://taichiforhealthinstitute.org/history-of-tai-chi-2/

[91] Jahnke R, Larkey L, Rogers C, Etnier J, Lin F. A comprehensive review of health benefits of qigong and tai chi. American Journal of Health Promotion. 2010;**24**(6):e1-e25

[92] Kong LJ, Lauche R, Klose P, Bu JH, Yang XC, Guo CQ, et al. Tai chi for chronic pain conditions: A systematic review and meta-analysis of randomized controlled trials. Scientific Reports [Internet]. 2016;**6**(1) Available from: https://www.nature.com/articles/srep25325

[93] Wells C, Kolt GS, Bialocerkowski A. Defining Pilates exercise: A systematic

review. Complementary Therapies in Medicine. 2012;**20**(4):253-262

[94] Theodoridou S, Iakovidis P, Lytras D, Kasimis K, Fetlis A, Kalitsiou K. Effect of pilates on the balance of older adults at high risk of falling: A narrative review. International Journal of Orthopaedics Sciences [Internet]. 2023;**9**(1):213-216. Available from: https://www.orthopaper.com/archives/2023/vol9issue1/PartD/9-1-42-494.pdf

Chapter 7

Impact of Physical Activity on Physical and Cognition Function among Community-Living Older Adults

Milan Chang Gudjonsson

Abstract

The aging population presents unique challenges to healthcare systems worldwide, particularly in terms of maintaining physical function and cognitive abilities in old age. Physical activity (PA) is emerging as a potent intervention to enhance the well-being and functional independence of older individuals. The current review chapter will focus on the effect of PA on physical and cognitive function to provide comprehensive understanding of the interplay among community-dwelling older adults. The review (1) overviews the positive impact of PA on physical functions, including muscle strength, endurance, balance, and cardiovascular health, elucidating how these benefits contribute to improved mobility and reduced risk of falls among older adults, and (2) explores also how regular PA is associated with the cognitive benefits, including its preventive or delaying effect of cognitive decline, enhancements in memory, attention, executive function, and overall cognitive vitality. It emphasizes the critical role of PA in enhancing the overall capacity on managing daily living of older adults and offers insights into effective strategies for promoting active and healthy aging. These knowledge and insights can also guide healthcare practitioners, policymakers, and researchers in developing and implementing effective strategies to promote PA and support healthy aging in older populations.

Keywords: physical activity, cognitive function, lifestyle, aging, physical function

1. Introduction

Aging is an inevitable process that every individual undergoes as they progress through life. The global demographic changes show a significant shift that the proportion of older adults (aged 60 and above) steadily increasing [1]. This demographic transition has caused a growing interest in healthy aging and age-related health challenges [2, 3]. This phenomenon is attributed to a combination of factors, including declining birth rates and advancements in healthcare, resulting in extended life expectancies [4]. This review chapter underscores the significant role of PA in enhancing the quality of life and functional independence of community-living older

IntechOpen

adults, illuminating the pathways through which it positively impacts both physical and cognitive functions. It calls for continued research and targeted interventions to harness the potential of PA as a cornerstone of healthy aging. This perspective sheds light on the following impact of an aging population on our society. The potential impact of an aging population on our society are followings:

1. Healthcare challenges: A significant increase in the older population presents various challenges for healthcare systems worldwide. There is a higher demand for healthcare services, particularly for age-related diseases and conditions such as Alzheimer's disease, diabetes, and cardiovascular problems.

2. Economic implications: The aging population can also have economic implications. As the older population grows, it may affect economic productivity and labor markets. Governments need to address these challenges to maintain economic stability.

3. Social considerations: An aging population can lead to changes in family structures and caregiving dynamics. The responsibility of caring for elderly family members often falls on the younger generation, impacting their work-life balance and overall well-being.

2. Understanding factors contributing to the increase of older population

Chronological aging refers to the passage of time as measured by one's date of birth [5], commonly used to determine an individual's age, wherein each passing year contributes to one's chronological age. Life expectancy (LE) is an important indicator for measuring the growth of the aging population [6], which is increasing globally as a result of reduced mortality among the older individuals [7]. Another significant factor contributing to the growth of the older population is the decline in birth rates observed in many countries [7, 8], resulting in a phenomenon known as "population aging." With fewer young people being born, the proportion of older individuals in the population naturally increases. Enhanced healthcare and medical advancements have also played a pivotal role in extending LE [9]. Medical conditions that were once fatal are now manageable or treatable, allowing individuals to lead longer and healthier lives. Improved accessibility to healthcare services and preventive measures has further contributed to this trend [10]. Moreover, economic stability and social welfare programs have provided support for older individuals [11], enabling them to lead more comfortable lives during their later years.

3. Impacts of PA on physical and cognitive function among older population

Physical and cognitive function are two fundamental aspects of an individual's well-being, influencing their ability to live independently and maintain a high quality of life (M. [12–14]). Aging-related functional decline can result in numerous health issues, reduced autonomy, decreased independence, and heightened pressure on healthcare systems [15, 16]. Given the importance of physical function and cognition in the lives of older adults, understanding how PA impacts these domains is crucial. The present chapter explores the current body of evidence on the topic, highlighting the potential benefits of regular PA on the physical and cognitive function of older adults.

Muscular strength declines 3% every year, and muscle mass reduces about 2% after 40 [17–20]. These phenomena of decline in both muscular strength and muscle mass with aging are well-known, and it is important to consider that the cause of this decline may not solely be attributed to the aging process itself but could also be linked to the reduction in PA that typically accompanies the aging process. Reduction in PA accelerated myoatrophy, which causes the loss of muscle mass and eventually lower basal metabolism [21, 22]. These changes lead to surplus energy increases and the accumulation of lipids [23, 24], which may further cause health problems, including higher blood pressure or blood glucose levels [25–27]. The significance of PA in maintaining our health has been long acknowledged. Regular PA offers numerous benefits, including (1) improving cardiovascular health, (2) enhancing or preserving cognitive and physical function [28, 29], and (3) reducing the risk of cognitive decline and major neurocognitive disorder among older adults [30, 31].

Clear evidences suggest that PA is beneficial for maintaining cognitive function, reducing risk of major neurocognitive disorder, and brain atrophy among older adults [30, 32]. While obesity and overweight were found to increase risk of major neurocognitive disorder [33], brain volumes (total brain tissue volume and gray matter and white matter volumes) are also strongly related to atherosclerosis [34], as well as to vascular risk factors such as systolic and diastolic blood pressure [35] or diabetes [36, 37]. The effect of regular PA and obesity on brain health may reflect lifestyle factors [32] or underlying modulation of neurotrophic and vascular risk factors as demonstrated in clinical and experimental research [38, 39].

4. Impact of PA on mobility and associated cognitive function

Those with low physical performance have a significantly higher risk of future institutionalization and disability onset [40–42]. While regular PA participation is linked with positive health outcomes, lack of PA has been also associated with increased disability and poor physical function among older adults [43]. Particularly, the mobility disability has been shown its predictive value for future institutionalization, mortality, and disability onset [40, 44]. Therefore, mobility function of older adults is often used as a clinical screening tool for the older population [43]. On the other hand, it is also suggested that those with low cognitive function have a lower mobility function compared with those with normal cognitive function (M. [12, 45, 46]). As the ability to move from one location to another is closely linked to factors such as attention, body coordination, and adaptability to one's surroundings [12, 47], older adults may need to maintain a higher level of cognitive function in order to sustain their independence in daily life.

5. Cognitive impairment among older adults

It is crucial to prioritize efforts to prevent or postpone cognitive decline in older adults [48]. Nevertheless, a substantial number of major neurocognitive disorder patients also experience damage from other vascular brain diseases, including mini-strokes, which are ranked as the fifth leading cause of death in the United States [49]. Earlier research has suggested that this major neurocognitive disorder could potentially rank as the third leading cause of death for older individuals, trailing only behind heart disease and cancer [50]. Memory problems are typically one of the first signs of cognitive impairment [51]. Some people with more memory problems than normal for their age may also have mild cognitive impairment (MCI), but their symptoms do not interfere with their everyday lives [52]. Movement difficulties and problems with the sense of smell have also been linked to MCI [53, 54].

While the impact of PA on cognitive functions is evident, several limitations need to be considered when interpreting the results. First, most studies had PA data collected close to the time at which cognitive function was assessed or major neurocognitive disorder diagnosed. With the short time intervals between PA and major neurocognitive disorder, it is difficult to determine whether the reported PA acts as a risk factor for cognitive decline or serves as an indicator of incipient disease. Second, most previous studies have examined either the relationship between PA and global cognitive performance or major neurocognitive disorder, but not both simultaneously. Third, studies that investigated the relationship between midlife PA and the risk of major neurocognitive disorder were mixed, and there is limited information on the association between levels of PA earlier in life and brain atrophy among older adults. At last, most studies investigating age-related changes in cerebral volume were cross-sectional and utilized small sample sizes of healthy older individuals or larger samples with all age groups. Further, longitudinal research on the impact of long-term PA on brain health is vital for a comprehensive understanding of these relationships.

While older people with MCI are at greater risk for developing major neurocognitive disorder, some may go back to normal cognition [53]. Researchers are studying biomarkers (biological signs of disease found in brain images, cerebrospinal fluid, and blood) to detect early sign in the brains of people with MCI and people with normal cognition who may be at greater risk for the major neurocognitive disorder [55]. Previous studies indicated that early detection is possible, but more research is needed before these medical techniques are available for the everyday medical practice to diagnose AD [48].

6. Effective PA intervention to prevent functional decline

Numerous exercise intervention studies have demonstrated that exercise improves physical performance in old age [12, 56, 57]. Further, regular PA or exercise also has a positive association with cognitive performance in the short- or long-term period [12, 58, 59]. Among various types of exercise for older adults, resistance exercise is one of the most feasible types of exercise to increase muscle mass and strength [59–61]. Particularly for the prevention of mobility disability and sarcopenia, the strength training is suggested as the most effective training method for older adults [59, 62, 63], even for those with limited mobility or cardiovascular fitness [64].

Cross-sectional studies have also shown that PA and physical performance are strongly associated with cognitive function [65–67], while it is possible that the improvement of physical performance by the exercise intervention may vary by baseline cognitive status [12]. Exercise intervention studies have primarily focused on investigating the improvement of physical performance and cognitive function among older adults following the intervention period [12, 13, 56, 62]. The specific findings related to the influence of various types of physical activity on cognitive function are as follows.

a. Engaging in regular aerobic exercises, such as running, swimming, or cycling, has been associated with improved cognitive functions, especially memory and attention, and has been correlated with increased hippocampal volume, contributing to memory enhancement and reduced cognitive decline risk [68–70].

b. Strength training, such as weightlifting or resistance exercises, has been found to benefit cognitive functions such as attention and memory [71]. Research suggests that resistance training can positively affect cognitive tasks and memory performance [59, 72, 73].

c. Activities, such as dance and coordination exercises, including tai chi, have been associated with improved cognitive functions related to praxis and visuospatial skills. Studies have shown that these activities can positively impact cognitive performance, particularly in the area of visuospatial abilities [74, 75]. Yoga and meditation practices have demonstrated significant benefits for attention and memory, with studies indicating that regular yoga practice can improve cognitive functions, including memory, attention, and processing speed [76, 77].

d. Certain cognitive training programs and brain games have been designed to target specific cognitive functions, including memory, attention, and language. Research suggests that engaging in these activities can lead to improvements in cognitive performance and function [78–80].

7. Other potentially modifiable risk factors for cognitive decline

Although age is the strongest risk factor for cognitive decline, major neurocognitive disorder may not be an inevitable consequence of aging [81, 82]. Several recent studies have shown that lifestyle-related risk factors, including physical inactivity, tobacco use, unhealthy diets, and harmful use of alcohol, are strongly associated with cognitive impairment and major neurocognitive disorder [83]. Hypertension, diabetes, hypercholesterolemia, obesity, and depression are all associated with an elevated risk of experiencing cognitive decline or developing major neurocognitive disorder [84, 85]. Other potentially modifiable risk factors, such as social isolation and cognitive inactivity, were also linked to the development of major neurocognitive disorder [48]. The risk reduction guidelines for cognitive decline and major neurocognitive disorder from WHO provide evidence-based guidance for a public health response to major neurocognitive disorder. These modifiable risk factors suggest that prevention of cognitive decline or major neurocognitive disorder is possible through a public health approach. Several evidence-based research have investigated whether reducing modifiable risk factors decrease the risk for major neurocognitive disorder [14, 86].

8. Types of intervention to prevent cognitive decline

Cognitive impairment and major neurocognitive disorder are complex, multifactorial disorders, and multi-domain interventions targeting several risk factors and disease mechanisms simultaneously could be needed for optimum preventive effects [85]. Previous prevention trials for cognitive impairment and major neurocognitive disorder have reported positive associations with cognition for PA, cognitive training,

Multimodal intervention programs: Implementing a long-term multicomponent program that combines various types of intervention including PA, cognitive training, social activity, and nutritional and cardiovascular counseling, has been shown to be effective in improving overall fitness, reducing sedentary behavior, and preventing a major neurocognitive disorder [85, 93].
Aerobic exercise programs: Implementing structured aerobic exercise programs, such as walking, jogging, or cycling, has shown significant effectiveness in reducing sedentary behavior and improving overall physical health. These programs are often tailored to individual fitness levels and can be conducted in group settings or individually [94–96].
Strength training interventions: Incorporating strength training interventions, including resistance exercises and weightlifting, has been found to be effective in promoting muscle strength, improving overall fitness, and combating the negative effects of a sedentary lifestyle, particularly in older adults [97].
Mind–body with flexibility and balance exercise programs: Interventions that integrate mind–body exercises, flexibility, and balance include tai-chi, yoga, and Pilates have demonstrated effectiveness in reducing sedentary behavior and promoting PA, while also providing benefits for mental well-being and stress reduction [74, 75, 77].

Table 1.
Effective types of intervention on cognition for older adults.

or both in smaller and shorter intervention studies [87–89]. Few prevention trials for cardiovascular disease and type 2 diabetes have emphasized the importance of a multi-domain approach [37, 87]. Multicomponent randomized controlled trials in individuals at risk of major neurocognitive disorder have been also recommended as an effective and feasible approach [85, 90]. Previous findings suggest that a risk factors other than genetics play a role in the development of AD [84]. One of a great deal of interest could be the relationship between cognitive decline and vascular conditions such as heart disease, stroke, and high blood pressure, as well as metabolic conditions, such as diabetes and obesity [91]. In general, a nutritious diet, PA, social engagement, and mentally stimulating pursuits have all been associated with helping people stay healthy as they age [90, 92]. These factors help in reducing the risk of cognitive decline [85]. However, evidence that short-term and single-component PA interventions promote cognitive function and prevent cognitive decline or major neurocognitive disorder in older adults is largely insufficient. Various forms of PA and exercise interventions have provided compelling evidence in countering sedentary habits and encouraging PA. These interventions include the followings (**Table 1**).

9. Impact of preventive intervention in adults with MCI

For cognitive outcomes in adults with MCI, evidence is still insufficient to indicate that PA interventions have a positive effect on cognition [31, 91]. However, these benefits are not consistent across all cognitive domains. This clinical trial proposal tests the efficacy and additive/synergistic effects of an exercise and cognitive training intervention on cognition with other risk factor management (social activity, nutrition, alcohol, and metabolic syndrome) in older adults who are diagnosed with MCI. Exercise and cognitive training are two promising interventions for preventing major neurocognitive disorders. Exercise increases fitness, which, in turn, improves brain structure and function, while cognitive training improves selective neural function intensively [48]. Various studies that tested cognitive training effects have reported discrepant findings due to varying programs [79, 98]. Hence, combined exercise and cognitive training may very well have an additive or synergistic effect on cognition by complementary strengthening of different neural functions. A meta-analysis of randomized controlled trials revealed a moderate effect of PA, with the most significant effect size observed for executive control processes [69, 99]. Optimal cognitive benefits were observed when aerobic training was combined with strength and flexibility training. Those review studies emphasized that a minimum of 30 minutes of PA training for over 6 months appeared necessary to establish stable cognitive effects in older adults. Moreover, the study suggested that engaging in moderate-intensity exercise, with an average duration of 1 hour per session, at least three times per week, could yield more pronounced cognitive and brain effects.

10. Conclusion

The impact of PA and exercise on physical function and cognition among community-living older adults is substantial. Regular PA and exercise have been proven to boost muscular strength, balance, mobility, cognitive function, and overall well-being in older population. The mechanisms underlying the positive impact of PA on physical function and cognition in older adults are multifaceted. Factors, such as increased blood flow to the brain, the release of neurotrophic factors, and reduced inflammation, contribute to these benefits. It is crucial for healthcare professionals, policymakers, and community organizations to facilitate initiatives that promote regular PA among older adults. This includes providing accessible exercise programs, educating about the benefits of PA and exercise, and establishing age-friendly environments. While existing literature highlights the positive relationship between PA, physical function, and cognition, further research is needed to fully understand this complex association. Long-term randomized controlled trials and investigations into the most effective types and intensities of exercise for different older adult populations can offer valuable insights.

Highlighting PA as an essential component of healthy aging is crucial, and continuous research in this area will further inform strategies aimed at improving the lives of older adults globally. As societies age, investing in older adults' health through PA initiatives will help to promote a healthier and more dynamic future for all.

Author details

Milan Chang Gudjonsson
Icelandic Gerontological Research Institute, University Hospital of Iceland, Iceland

*Address all correspondence to: changmilan@gmail.com

References

[1] United Nations. World Population Prospects: The 2017 Revision, Multimedia Library. United Nations Department of Economic and Social Affairs; 2017. pp. 1-8. Available from: https://www.un.org/development/desa/publications/world-population-prospects-the-2017-revision.html

[2] Beard JR, Officer A, de Carvalho IA, Sadana R, Pot AM, Michel J-P, et al. The world report on ageing and health: A policy framework for healthy ageing. Lancet (London, England). 2016;**387**(10033):2145-2154. DOI: 10.1016/S0140-6736(15)00516-4

[3] World Health Organization. Risk Reduction of Cognitive Decline and Dementia: WHO Guidelines. WHO; 2019b:12-43. Available from: https://www.who.int/publications/i/item/9789241550543

[4] Knudsen AK, Allebeck P, Tollånes MC, Skogen JC, Iburg KM, McGrath JJ, et al. Life expectancy and disease burden in the Nordic countries: Results from the global burden of diseases, injuries, and risk factors study 2017. The Lancet Public Health. 2019;**4**(12):e658-e669. DOI: 10.1016/S2468-2667(19)30224-5

[5] Han LK, Verhoeven JE, Tyrka AR, Penninx BW, Wolkowitz OM, Månsson KN, et al. Accelerating research on biological aging and mental health: Current challenges and future directions. Psychoneuroendocrinology. 2019;**106**:293-311. DOI: 10.1016/j.psyneuen.2019.04.004

[6] Christensen K, Doblhammer G, Rau R, Vaupel JW. Ageing populations: The challenges ahead. Lancet. 2009;**374**(9696):1196-1208. DOI: 10.1016/S0140-6736(09)61460-4

[7] Ouellette N, Barbieri M, Wilmoth JR. Period-based mortality change: Turning points in trends since 1950. Population and Development Review. 2014;**40**(1):77-106. DOI: 10.1111/j.1728-4457.2014.00651.x

[8] United Nations. The Problem with 'Too Few'. United Nations Population Fund; 2023. Available from: https://www.unfpa.org/swp2023/too-few

[9] World Health Organization. Healthy Life Expectancy (HALE) at Age 60 (Years). The Global Health Observatory Explore a World of Health Data. 2020. Available from: https://www.who.int/data/gho/data/indicators/indicator-details/GHO/gho-ghe-hale-healthy-life-expectancy-at-age-60

[10] Hao L, Xu X, Dupre ME, Guo A, Zhang X, Qiu L, et al. Adequate access to healthcare and added life expectancy among older adults in China. BMC Geriatrics. 2020;**20**(1):129. DOI: 10.1186/s12877-020-01524-9

[11] World Health Organization. Health and social care near the end of life: can policies reduce costs and improve outcomes? Economics of Ageing. WHO; 2019a. Available from: https://iris.who.int/bitstream/handle/10665/349803/Policy-brief-1997-8073-2021-1-eng.pdf?sequence=1

[12] Chang M. The effect of cognitive function on mobility improvement among community-living older adults: A 12-week resistance exercise intervention study. Aging, Neuropsychology, and Cognition. 2019;**27**(3):385-396. DOI: 10.1080/13825585.2019.1623167

[13] Chang M, Geirsdottir OG, Eymundsdottir H, Thorsdottir I,

Jonsson PV, Ramel A. Association between baseline handgrip strength and cognitive function assessed before and after a 12-week resistance exercise intervention among community-living older adults. Aging and Health Research. 2022;**2**(3):100092. DOI: 10.1016/j.ahr.2022.100092

[14] Komulainen P, Tuomilehto J, Savonen K, Männikkö R, Hassinen M, Lakka TA, et al. Exercise, diet, and cognition in a 4-year randomized controlled trial: Dose-responses to exercise training (DR's EXTRA). The American Journal of Clinical Nutrition. 2021;**113**(6):1428-1439. DOI: 10.1093/ajcn/nqab018

[15] Oude Voshaar RC, Jeuring HW, Borges MK, van den Brink RHS, Marijnissen RM, Hoogendijk EO, et al. Course of frailty stratified by physical and mental multimorbidity patterns: A 5-year follow-up of 92,640 participants of the LifeLines cohort study. BMC Medicine. 2021;**19**:29. DOI: 10.1186/s12916-021-01904-x

[16] Wang T, Wu Y, Li W, Li S, Sun Y, Li S, et al. Weak grip strength and cognition predict functional limitation in older Europeans. Journal of the American Geriatrics Society. 2019;**67**(1):93-99. DOI: 10.1111/jgs.15611

[17] Chiles Shaffer N, Fabbri E, Ferrucci L, Shardell M, Simonsick EM, Studenski S. Muscle quality, strength, and lower extremity physical performance in the Baltimore longitudinal study of aging. The Journal of Frailty & Aging. 2017;**6**(4):183-187. DOI: 10.14283/jfa.2017.24

[18] Goodpaster BH, Park SW, Harris TB, Kritchevsky SB, Nevitt M, Schwartz AV, et al. The loss of skeletal muscle strength, mass, and quality in older adults: The health, aging and body composition study. The Journals of Gerontology. Series A, Biological Sciences and Medical Sciences. 2006;**61**(10):1059-1064. DOI: 10.1093/gerona/61.10.1059

[19] Visser M, Goodpaster BH, Kritchevsky SB, Newman AB, Nevitt M, Rubin SM, et al. Muscle mass, muscle strength, and muscle fat infiltration as predictors of incident mobility limitations in well-functioning older persons. The Journals of Gerontology. Series A, Biological Sciences and Medical Sciences. 2005;**60**(3):324-333

[20] von Haehling S, Morley JE, Anker SD. An overview of sarcopenia: Facts and numbers on prevalence and clinical impact. Journal of Cachexia, Sarcopenia and Muscle. 2010;**1**(2):129-133. DOI: 10.1007/s13539-010-0014-2

[21] Liu CK, Leng X, Hsu F-C, Kritchevsky SB, Ding J, Earnest CP, et al. The impact of sarcopenia on a physical activity intervention: The lifestyle interventions and independence for elders pilot study (LIFE-P). The Journal of Nutrition, Health & Aging. 2014;**18**(1):59-64. DOI: 10.1007/s12603-013-0369-0

[22] Steffl M, Bohannon RW, Sontakova L, Tufano JJ, Shiells K, Holmerova I. Relationship between sarcopenia and physical activity in older people: A systematic review and meta-analysis. Clinical Interventions in Aging. 2017;**12**:835-845. DOI: 10.2147/CIA.S132940

[23] Biolo G, Cederholm T, Muscaritoli M. Muscle contractile and metabolic dysfunction is a common feature of sarcopenia of aging and chronic diseases: From sarcopenic obesity to cachexia. Clinical Nutrition. 2014;**33**(5):737-748. DOI: 10.1016/j.clnu.2014.03.007

[24] Botoseneanu A, Chen H, Ambrosius WT, Allore HG,

Anton S, Folta SC, et al. Effect of metabolic syndrome on the mobility benefit of a structured physical activity intervention—The lifestyle interventions and Independence for elders randomized clinical trial. Journal of the American Geriatrics Society. 2017;**65, 6**:1244-1250. DOI: 10.1111/jgs.14793

[25] Kowal P, Charlton K. Joint effect of mid- and late-life blood pressure on the brain: The AGES-Reykjavik study. Neurology. 2015;**84**(3):329. DOI: 10.1212/01.wnl.0000460552.36620.a9

[26] Schubert CM, Rogers NL, Remsberg KE, Sun SS, Chumlea WC, Demerath EW, et al. Lipids, lipoproteins, lifestyle, adiposity and fat-free mass during middle age: The Fels longitudinal study. International Journal of Obesity. 2006;**30**(2):251-260. DOI: 10.1038/sj.ijo.0803129

[27] Zhou B, Perel P, Mensah GA, Ezzati M. Global epidemiology, health burden and effective interventions for elevated blood pressure and hypertension. Nature Reviews. Cardiology. 2021;**18**(11):785-802. DOI: 10.1038/s41569-021-00559-8

[28] Best JR, Davis JC, Liu-Ambrose T. Longitudinal analysis of physical performance, functional status, physical activity, and mood in relation to executive function in older adults who fall. Journal of the American Geriatrics Society. 2015;**63**(6):1112-1120. DOI: 10.1111/jgs.13444

[29] Pahor M, Guralnik JM, Ambrosius WT, Blair S, Bonds DE, Church TS, et al. Effect of structured physical activity on prevention of major mobility disability in older adults: The LIFE study randomized clinical trial. JAMA. 2014;**311**(23):2387-2396. DOI: 10.1001/jama.2014.5616

[30] Bherer L, Erickson KI, Liu-Ambrose T. A review of the effects of physical activity and exercise on cognitive and brain functions in older adults. Journal of Aging Research. 2013;**2013**:657508. DOI: 10.1155/2013/657508

[31] Brasure M, Desai P, Davila H, Nelson VA, Calvert C, Jutkowitz E, et al. Physical activity interventions in preventing cognitive decline and Alzheimer-type dementia: A systematic review. Annals of Internal Medicine. 2018;**168**(1):30-38. DOI: 10.7326/M17-1528

[32] Hopstock LA, Deraas TS, Henriksen A, Martiny-Huenger T, Grimsgaard S. Changes in adiposity, physical activity, cardiometabolic risk factors, diet, physical capacity and well-being in inactive women and men aged 57-74 years with obesity and cardiovascular risk – A 6-month complex lifestyle intervention with 6-month follow-up. PLoS One. 2021;**16**(8):e0256631. DOI: 10.1371/journal.pone.0256631

[33] Lee CM, Woodward M, Batty GD, Beiser AS, Bell S, Berr C, et al. Association of anthropometry and weight change with risk of dementia and its major subtypes: A meta-analysis consisting 2.8 million adults with 57 294 cases of dementia. Obesity Reviews. 2020;**21**(4):e12989. DOI: 10.1111/obr.12989

[34] Miyashita M, Stensel DJ, Burns SF, Sasai H, Tanaka K. The effects of 30 min of exercise on cardiovascular disease risk factors in healthy and obese individuals. Atherosclerosis. 2011;**216**(2):496-497. DOI: 10.1016/j.atherosclerosis.2011.02.001

[35] Sasai H, Sairenchi T, Irie F, Otaka E, Iso H, Tanaka K, et al.

Long-term exposure to elevated blood pressure and mortality from cardiovascular disease in a Japanese population: The Ibaraki prefectural health study. Hypertension Research. 2011;**34**(1):139-144. DOI: 10.1038/hr.2010.173

[36] Francois ME, Durrer C, Pistawka KJ, Halperin FA, Little JP. Resistance-based interval exercise acutely improves endothelial function in type 2 diabetes. American Journal of Physiology - Heart and Circulatory Physiology. 2016;**311**(5):H1258-H1267. DOI: 10.1152/ajpheart.00398.2016

[37] Gæde P, Lund-Andersen H, Parving H-H, Pedersen O. Effect of a multifactorial intervention on mortality in type 2 diabetes. New England Journal of Medicine. 2008;**358**(6):580-591. DOI: 10.1056/NEJMoa0706245

[38] Arai AE. New insights from major prospective cohort studies with cardiovascular magnetic resonance (CMR). Current Cardiology Reports. 2015;**17**(6):46. DOI: 10.1007/s11886-015-0599-3

[39] Heitmann KA, Welde B, Løchen M-L, Stylidis M, Schirmer H, Morseth B. Longitudinal associations between cumulative physical activity and change in structure and function of the left side of the heart: The Tromsø study 2007-2016. Frontiers in Cardiovascular Medicine. 2022;**9**:882077. Available from: https://www.frontiersin.org/articles/10.3389/fcvm.2022.882077

[40] Guralnik JM, Ferrucci L, Pieper CF, Leveille SG, Markides KS, Ostir GV, et al. Lower extremity function and subsequent disability consistency across studies, predictive models, and value of gait speed alone compared with the short physical performance battery. The Journals of Gerontology Series A: Biological Sciences and Medical Sciences. 2000;**55**(4):M221-M231. DOI: 10.1093/gerona/55.4.M221

[41] Ostir GV, Berges IM, Ottenbacher KJ, Fisher SR, Barr E, Hebel JR, et al. Gait speed and dismobility in older adults. Archives of Physical Medicine and Rehabilitation. 2015;**96**(9):1641-1645. DOI: 10.1016/j.apmr.2015.05.017

[42] Vita AJ, Terry RB, Hubert HB, Fries JF. Aging, health risks, and cumulative disability. The New England Journal of Medicine. 1998;**338**(15):1035-1041. DOI: 10.1056/NEJM199804093381506

[43] Studenski SA, Peters KW, Alley DE, Cawthon PM, McLean RR, Harris TB, et al. The FNIH sarcopenia project: Rationale, study description, conference recommendations, and final estimates. The Journals of Gerontology: Series A. 2014;**69**(5):547-558. DOI: 10.1093/gerona/glu010

[44] Guralnik JM, Ferrucci L, Simonsick EM, Salive ME, Wallace RB. Lower-extremity function in persons over the age of 70 years as a predictor of subsequent disability. New England Journal of Medicine. 1995;**332**(9):556-562. DOI: 10.1056/NEJM199503023320902

[45] Eggermont LH, Gavett BE, Volkers KM, Blankevoort CG, Scherder EJ, Jefferson AL, et al. Lower-extremity function in cognitively healthy aging, mild cognitive impairment, and Alzheimer's disease. Archives of Physical Medicine and Rehabilitation. 2010;**91**(4):584-588. DOI: 10.1016/j.apmr.2009.11.020

[46] Raji MA, Al Snih S, Ostir GV, Markides KS, Ottenbacher KJ. Cognitive status and future risk of frailty

in older Mexican Americans. The Journals of Gerontology: Series A. 2010;**65A**(11):1228-1234. DOI: 10.1093/gerona/glq121

[47] Buchman AS, Boyle PA, Leurgans SE, Barnes LL, Bennett DA. Cognitive function is associated with the development of mobility impairments in community-dwelling elders. The American Journal of Geriatric Psychiatry. 2011;**19**(6):571-580. DOI: 10.1097/JGP.0b013e3181ef7a2e

[48] Livingston G, Huntley J, Sommerlad A, Ames D, Ballard C, Banerjee S, et al. Dementia prevention, intervention, and care: 2020 report of the lancet commission. Lancet (London, England). 2020;**396**(10248):413-446. DOI: 10.1016/S0140-6736(20)30367-6

[49] Alzheimer's disease facts and figures, Alzheimer's & Dementia, 2023;**19**(4):1598-1695. DOI: 10.1002/alz.13016

[50] Weuve J, Hebert LE, Scherr PA, Evans DA. Deaths in the United States among persons with Alzheimer's disease (2010-2050). Alzheimer's & Dementia: The Journal of the Alzheimer's Association. 2014;**10**(2):e40-e46. DOI: 10.1016/j.jalz.2014.01.004

[51] Ryu SY, Lee SB, Kim TW, Lee TJ. Subjective memory complaints, depressive symptoms and instrumental activities of daily living in mild cognitive impairment. International Psychogeriatrics. 2016;**28**(3):487-494. DOI: 10.1017/S1041610215001945

[52] Lenehan ME, Klekociuk SZ, Summers MJ. Absence of a relationship between subjective memory complaint and objective memory impairment in mild cognitive impairment (MCI): Is it time to abandon subjective memory complaint as an MCI diagnostic criterion? International Psychogeriatrics. 2012;**24**(9):1505-1514. DOI: 10.1017/S1041610212000695

[53] Butler M, McCreedy E, Nelson VA, Desai P, Ratner E, Fink HA, et al. Does cognitive training prevent cognitive decline?: A systematic review. Annals of Internal Medicine. 2018;**168**(1):63-68. DOI: 10.7326/M17-1531

[54] Farias ST, Lau K, Harvey D, Denny K, Barba C, Mefford AN. Early functional limitations in cognitively normal older adults predicts diagnostic conversion to mild cognitive impairment. Journal of the American Geriatrics Society. 2017;**65**(6):1152-1158. DOI: 10.1111/jgs.14835

[55] Liang J-H, Xu Y, Lin L, Jia R-X, Zhang H-B, Hang L. Comparison of multiple interventions for older adults with Alzheimer disease or mild cognitive impairment: A PRISMA-compliant network meta-analysis. Medicine. 2018;**97**(20):e10744. DOI: 10.1097/MD.0000000000010744

[56] Eriksen CS, Garde E, Reislev NL, Wimmelmann CL, Bieler T, Ziegler AK, et al. Physical activity as intervention for age-related loss of muscle mass and function: Protocol for a randomised controlled trial (the LISA study). BMJ Open. 2016;**6**(12):e012951. DOI: 10.1136/bmjopen-2016-012951

[57] Gill TM, Pahor M, Guralnik JM, McDermott MM, King AC, Buford TW, et al. Effect of structured physical activity on prevention of serious fall injuries in adults aged 70-89: Randomized clinical trial (LIFE study). BMJ. 2016;**352**:i245. DOI: 10.1136/bmj.i245

[58] Chang M. The effect of midlife physical activity on cognitive function among older adults: AGES—Reykjavik

study. The Journals of Gerontology: Series A. 2010;**65**(12):1369-1374. DOI: 10.1093/gerona/glq152

[59] Chang Y-K, Pan C-Y, Chen F-T, Tsai C-L, Huang C-C. Effect of resistance-exercise training on cognitive function in healthy older adults: A review. Journal of Aging and Physical Activity. 2012a;**20**(4):497-517

[60] Mavros Y, Gates N, Wilson GC, Jain N, Meiklejohn J, Brodaty H, et al. Mediation of cognitive function improvements by strength gains after resistance training in older adults with mild cognitive impairment: Outcomes of the study of mental and resistance training. Journal of the American Geriatrics Society. 2017;**65**(3):550-559. DOI: 10.1111/jgs.14542

[61] Snijders T, Leenders M, de Groot LCPGM, van Loon LJC, Verdijk LB. Muscle mass and strength gains following 6 months of resistance type exercise training are only partly preserved within one year with autonomous exercise continuation in older adults. Experimental Gerontology. 2019;**121**:71-78. DOI: 10.1016/j.exger.2019.04.002

[62] Aartolahti E, Lönnroos E, Hartikainen S, Häkkinen A. Long-term strength and balance training in prevention of decline in muscle strength and mobility in older adults. Aging Clinical and Experimental Research. 2020;**32**(1):59-66. DOI: 10.1007/s40520-019-01155-0

[63] Reid KF, Martin KI, Doros G, Clark DJ, Hau C, Patten C, et al. Comparative effects of light or heavy resistance power training for improving lower extremity power and physical performance in mobility-limited older adults. The Journals of Gerontology. Series A, Biological Sciences and Medical Sciences. 2015;**70**(3):374-380. DOI: 10.1093/gerona/glu156

[64] Billot M, Calvani R, Urtamo A, Sánchez-Sánchez JL, Ciccolari-Micaldi C, Chang M, et al. Preserving mobility in older adults with physical frailty and sarcopenia: Opportunities, challenges, and recommendations for physical activity interventions. Clinical Interventions in Aging. 2020;**15**:1675-1690. DOI: 10.2147/CIA.S253535

[65] Boisvert-Vigneault K, Payette H, Audet M, Gaudreau P, Bélanger M, Dionne IJ. Relationships between physical activity across lifetime and health outcomes in older adults: Results from the NuAge cohort. Preventive Medicine. 2016;**91**:37-42. DOI: 10.1016/j.ypmed.2016.07.018

[66] Gu Y, Beato JM, Amarante E, Chesebro AG, Manly JJ, Schupf N, et al. Assessment of leisure time physical activity and brain health in a multiethnic cohort of older adults. JAMA Network Open. 2020;**3**(11):e2026506. DOI: 10.1001/jamanetworkopen.2020.26506

[67] Jang JY, Kim J. Association between handgrip strength and cognitive impairment in elderly Koreans: A population-based cross-sectional study. Journal of Physical Therapy Science. 2015;**27**(12):3911-3915. DOI: 10.1589/jpts.27.3911

[68] Erickson KI, Voss MW, Prakash RS, Basak C, Szabo A, Chaddock L, et al. Exercise training increases size of hippocampus and improves memory. Proceedings of the National Academy of Sciences. 2011;**108**(7):3017-3022. DOI: 10.1073/pnas.1015950108

[69] Kramer AF, Erickson KI, McAuley E. Effects of physical activity on cognition and brain. In: Cognitive

Neurorehabilitation. Vol. 417. Cambridge University Press; 2008. pp. 417-434

[70] Yu F, Vock DM, Zhang L, Salisbury D, Nelson NW, Chow LS, et al. Cognitive effects of aerobic exercise in Alzheimer's disease: A pilot randomized controlled trial. Journal of Alzheimer's Disease. 2021;**80**(1):233-244. DOI: 10.3233/JAD-201100

[71] Venezia AC, Barney P, Spagnoli D, Greco-Hiranaka C, Piepmeier AT, Smith JC, et al. The effects of acute resistance exercise on memory, processing speed, and mood state after a cognitive challenge. Journal of Strength and Conditioning Research. 2023;**37**(9):1738-1745. DOI: 10.1519/JSC.0000000000004455

[72] Cassilhas RC, Viana VAR, Grassmann V, Santos RT, Santos RF, Tufik S, et al. The impact of resistance exercise on the cognitive function of the elderly. Medicine and Science in Sports and Exercise. 2007;**39**(8):1401-1407. DOI: 10.1249/mss.0b013e318060111f

[73] Loprinzi PD, Frith E, Edwards MK, Sng E, Ashpole N. The effects of exercise on memory function among young to middle-aged adults: Systematic review and recommendations for future research. American Journal of Health Promotion: AJHP. 2018;**32**(3):691-704. DOI: 10.1177/0890117117737409

[74] Zhang Y, Li C, Zou L, Liu X, Song W. The effects of mind-body exercise on cognitive performance in elderly: A systematic review and meta-analysis. International Journal of Environmental Research and Public Health. 2018;**15**(12):2791. DOI: 10.3390/ijerph15122791

[75] Zou L, Loprinzi PD, Yeung AS, Zeng N, Huang T. The beneficial effects of mind-body exercises for people with mild cognitive impairment: A systematic review with meta-analysis. Archives of Physical Medicine and Rehabilitation. 2019;**100**(8):1556-1573. DOI: 10.1016/j.apmr.2019.03.009

[76] Chobe S, Chobe M, Metri K, Patra SK, Nagaratna R. Impact of yoga on cognition and mental health among elderly: A systematic review. Complementary Therapies in Medicine. 2020;**52**:102421. DOI: 10.1016/j.ctim.2020.102421

[77] Gothe N, Pontifex MB, Hillman C, McAuley E. The acute effects of yoga on executive function. Journal of Physical Activity & Health. 2013;**10**(4):488-495. DOI: 10.1123/jpah.10.4.488

[78] Anguera J, Boccanfuso J, Rintoul J, Claflin O, Faraji F, Janowich J, et al. Video game training enhances cognitive control in older adults. Nature. 2013;**501**:97-101. DOI: 10.1038/nature12486

[79] Hill NTM, Mowszowski L, Naismith SL, Chadwick VL, Valenzuela M, Lampit A. Computerized cognitive training in older adults with mild cognitive impairment or dementia: A systematic review and meta-analysis. The American Journal of Psychiatry. 2017;**174**(4):329-340. DOI: 10.1176/appi.ajp.2016.16030360

[80] Lampit A, Hallock H, Valenzuela M. Computerized cognitive training in cognitively healthy older adults: A systematic review and meta-analysis of effect modifiers. PLoS Medicine. 2014;**11**(11):e1001756. DOI: 10.1371/journal.pmed.1001756

[81] Sperling RA, Aisen PS, Beckett LA, Bennett DA, Craft S, Fagan AM, et al. Toward defining the preclinical stages of Alzheimer's disease: Recommendations from the National Institute on Aging-Alzheimer's association workgroups on

diagnostic guidelines for Alzheimer's disease. Alzheimer's & Dementia. 2011;**7**(3):280-292. DOI: 10.1016/j.jalz.2011.03.003

[82] Winblad B, Amouyel P, Andrieu S, Ballard C, Brayne C, Brodaty H, et al. Defeating Alzheimer's disease and other dementias: A priority for European science and society. The Lancet Neurology. 2016;**15**(5):455-532. DOI: 10.1016/S1474-4422(16)00062-4

[83] Jack CR, Albert MS, Knopman DS, McKhann GM, Sperling RA, Carrillo MC, et al. Introduction to the recommendations from the National Institute on Aging-Alzheimer's association workgroups on diagnostic guidelines for Alzheimer's disease. Alzheimer's & Dementia. 2011;**7**(3):257-262. DOI: 10.1016/j.jalz.2011.03.004

[84] Frankish H, Horton R. Prevention and management of dementia: A priority for public health. The Lancet. 2017;**390**(10113):2614-2615. DOI: 10.1016/S0140-6736(17)31756-7

[85] Ngandu T, Lehtisalo J, Solomon A, Levälahti E, Ahtiluoto S, Antikainen R, et al. A 2 year multidomain intervention of diet, exercise, cognitive training, and vascular risk monitoring versus control to prevent cognitive decline in at-risk elderly people (FINGER): A randomised controlled trial. Lancet (London, England). 2015;**385**(9984):2255-2263. DOI: 10.1016/S0140-6736(15)60461-5

[86] Kivipelto M, Solomon A, Ahtiluoto S, Ngandu T, Lehtisalo J, Antikainen R, et al. The Finnish geriatric intervention study to prevent cognitive impairment and disability (FINGER): Study design and progress. Alzheimer's & Dementia: The Journal of the Alzheimer's Association. 2013;**9**(6):657-665. DOI: 10.1016/j.jalz.2012.09.012

[87] Fiatarone Singh MA, Gates N, Saigal N, Wilson GC, Meiklejohn J, Brodaty H, et al. The study of mental and resistance training (SMART) study—Resistance training and/or cognitive training in mild cognitive impairment: A randomized, double-blind, double-sham controlled trial. Journal of the American Medical Directors Association. 2014;**15**(12):873-880. DOI: 10.1016/j.jamda.2014.09.010

[88] O'Hara R, Brooks JO, Friedman L, Schröder CM, Morgan KS, Kraemer HC. Long-term effects of mnemonic training in community-dwelling older adults. Journal of Psychiatric Research. 2007;**41**(7):585-590. DOI: 10.1016/j.jpsychires.2006.04.010

[89] Smith PJ, Blumenthal JA, Hoffman BM, Cooper H, Strauman TA, Welsh-Bohmer K, et al. Aerobic exercise and neurocognitive performance: A meta-analytic review of randomized controlled trials. Psychosomatic Medicine. 2010;**72**(3):239-252. DOI: 10.1097/PSY.0b013e3181d14633

[90] Williams JW, Plassman BL, Burke J, Benjamin S. Preventing Alzheimer's disease and cognitive decline. Evidence Report/Technology Assessment. 2010;**193**:1-727

[91] Horr T, Messinger-Rapport B, Pillai JA. Systematic review of strengths and limitations of randomized controlled trials for non-pharmacological interventions in mild cognitive impairment: Focus on Alzheimer's disease. The Journal of Nutrition, Health & Aging. 2015;**19**(2):141-153. DOI: 10.1007/s12603-014-0565-6

[92] Sink KM, Espeland MA, Castro CM, Church T, Cohen R, Dodson JA, et al. Effect of a 24-month physical activity intervention vs health education

on cognitive outcomes in sedentary older adults: The LIFE randomized trial. JAMA. 2015;**314**(8):781-790. DOI: 10.1001/jama.2015.9617

[93] Sugimoto T, Sakurai T, Akatsu H, Doi T, Fujiwara Y, Hirakawa A, et al. The Japan-multimodal intervention trial for prevention of dementia (J-MINT): The study protocol for an 18-month, multicenter, randomized, controlled trial. The Journal of Prevention of Alzheimer's Disease. 2021;**8**(4):465-476. DOI: 10.14283/jpad.2021.29

[94] Baker LD, Frank LL, Foster-Schubert K, Green PS, Wilkinson CW, McTiernan A, et al. Effects of aerobic exercise on mild cognitive impairment. Archives of Neurology. 2010;**67**(1):71-79. DOI: 10.1001/archneurol.2009.307

[95] Kramer AF, Erickson KI. Capitalizing on cortical plasticity: Influence of physical activity on cognition and brain function. Trends in Cognitive Sciences. 2007;**11**(8):342-348. DOI: 10.1016/j.tics.2007.06.009

[96] Li L, Zhang S, Cui J, Chen L-Z, Wang X, Fan M, et al. Fitness-dependent effect of acute aerobic exercise on executive function. Frontiers in Physiology. 2019;**10**:902. DOI: 10.3389/fphys.2019.00902

[97] Alfaro-Acha A, Snih SA, Raji MA, Kuo Y-F, Markides KS, Ottenbacher KJ. Handgrip strength and cognitive decline in older Mexican Americans. The Journals of Gerontology. Series A, Biological Sciences and Medical Sciences. 2006;**61**(8):859-865

[98] Kane RL, Butler M, Fink HA, Brasure M, Davila H, Desai P, et al. Interventions to prevent age-related cognitive decline. In: Mild Cognitive Impairment, and Clinical Alzheimer's-Type Dementia. US: Agency for Healthcare Research and Quality; 2017. Available from: https://www.ncbi.nlm.nih.gov/sites/books/NBK442425/

[99] Erickson KI, Weinstein AM, Lopez OL. Physical activity, brain plasticity, and Alzheimer's disease. Archives of Medical Research. 2012;**43**(8):615-621. DOI: 10.1016/j.arcmed.2012.09.008